MEDICAL
TERMINOLOGY

THE BEST AND MOST EFFECTIVE WAY TO MEMORIZE, PRONOUNCE AND UNDERSTAND MEDICAL TERMS

Second Edition

DAVID ANDERSSON

Contents

Contents

Introduction

I want to thank you and congratulate you for buying the book, *"Medical Terminology: The Best and Most Effective Way to Memorize, Pronounce and Understand Medical Terms"*.

What did the doctor say? What did the patient say? What did the professor say? What's going on?

These are only few of the questions that people ask when faced with jargon-filled medical conversation in hospitals, schools, clinics, homes, and even at work. This book contains proven steps and strategies on how to understand, pronounce, and memorize medical terms, by using various methods. It also has tips and strategies to help you apply these methods.

Thanks again for buying this book, I hope you enjoy it!

Chapter 1:

The Importance of Learning Medical Terms

Medical terminology is the language used by medical professionals worldwide. It is universal to the medical and healthcare industry as it helps providers to completely understand what help a patient needs, or what is happening to the patient. It is important for nurses, doctors, other medical professionals, and medical students to be familiar with this language. Nowadays, with new medical professionals entering the industry, such as medical coders or transcriptionists and medical billers, learning medical terms is even more important. There is a high risk of improper management due to miscommunication between medical workers and patients, which can occur if workers do not know or use the correct medical terms.

At home or in clinics, knowing the right medical terms can prevent confusion and panic. Individuals who are familiar with medical terms can better understand their doctor and other medical professionals, especially in cases where medical procedures are required. In schools or universities, a better knowledge of medical terms can help students pass their exams.

In hospitals and in the medical field in general, medical terms make clinical proceedings easier because medical professionals can understand each others jargon. This works better for the patient's benefit, as it allows every person involved in the process of care to carry out their duties more efficiently.

> " Doctors often use different medical terms interchangeably. Depending on the context and situation, the terms could have different definitions.

Medical terms accurately describe the treatment that patients need to undergo and the conditions that they suffer from. Without proper knowledge of terms, communication between medical professionals may get confusing and in the end, patients might not get proper treatment. This would show that medical professionals are no longer effective in their job. Understanding medical terms, using them properly, and knowing their context has its benefits.

A. Benefits of Learning Medical Terms

1. It avoids medical errors.

Not properly documenting patients' medical records can get medical professionals in trouble. It can even put patients at bigger health risks. Medical records contain details that can help medical professionals diagnose patients more accurately, and thereby provide them with the right treatment. These records are packed with medical terms that help describe medical history of patients. For example, a doctor can avoid using certain medication on a particular patient if it is known from the patient's medical records that the patient has had a history of adverse allergic reactions to those drugs.

According to two major studies by the National Academy of Medicine, there are 44,000 to 98,000 deaths each year due to medical errors. These medical errors can range from wrong-site surgery and surgical injuries, improper transfusions and adverse drug events, restraint-related injuries or death, mistaken patient identities, falls, pressure ulcers, burns, and suicides. Another medical error, medication error, has emerged within the past 15 years and it claims around 7,000 deaths each year.

If all medical professionals receive proper medical terminology training, these deaths can be avoided.

2. It provides easy documentation and standardized communication.

Most of the time, medical terms are represented by abbreviations, which are used in medical records for documentation. Abbreviations are used because, if medical terms are translated into laymen's terms, documentation can become laborious. Fortunately, medical terms are standard, and therefore, can be understood by all medical professionals, even when they are in abbreviations.

3. It provides accurate diagnosis.

Standardized medical terms also help medical professionals understand their patients' medical condition. This helps them interpret complex information, and enables them to diagnose patients more accurately. It basically helps them answer the following questions:

- » Why is the patient seeking medical help?
- » What kind of treatment and care is needed to help the patient?

Being in, and studying for the medical industry has many benefits. It also has a lot of responsibilities and one of these is to learn, understand, and pronounce medical terms properly.

Chapter 2:

Understanding Medical Terms

Medical terms may seem like a foreign language at first glance. The words are usually long and can be confusing. The key to understanding such terms is to focus on their components, specifically on their prefixes, roots, and suffixes. The list of medical terms is very long. Knowing the meaning of only a few components can help understand and interpret a long list of medical terms. Let's figure out how this is done.

A. Break Long Words Apart

Majority of medical terms are made up of multiple parts. Breaking them apart makes it easier to understand single, long words. Long medical words consist of the following components:

Beginning	Middle	Ending
prefix	root	suffix
can be about shape, size, direction, or color	is often part of the body	can be about the same thing as the beginning, or it can be about a test or it can describe a problem

A good example of a medical term to break apart is:

Transesophageal   Echocardiogram

Trans	esophag	Eal		Echo	car-dio	gram
begin-ning (or prefix)	middle (or root)	ending (or suffix)		begin-ning (or prefix)	mid-dle (or root)	end-ing (or suffix)

Medical terms do not necessarily have a beginning or ending. Sometimes parts of words appear in different components or places. For example, the word cardio used in the example above, is also in the medical terms myocardial and cardiologist, though they appear in different places. Why and how this happens will be discussed in detail later.

B. Be Familiarized with Beginnings and Endings

Beginnings and endings vary in purpose and use. Here are some of the most commonly used words for medical terms beginnings and endings:

Purpose	Beginning/Ending Words	Description
About size	Macro	large
	Micro	small
	Megalo or megaly	Very large
About where	Peri	around
	Trans	across
	Endo	within or inside
	Inter	between

Chapter 2: Understanding Medical Terms

About color	Chloro	Green
	Leuk	White
	Eryth	Red
	Cyan	Blue
About problems	Dys	not working correctly/ normally
	Mal	Bad
	Emia	blood condition
	Itis	Inflammation
	Osis	condition or disease (usually non-inflammatory)
	Pathy	Disease
General use	Hyper	above normal
	Hypo	below normal
	Tachy	Fast
	Brady	slow

Some of commonly used beginnings and endings about tests and procedures:

Purpose	Words	Description
		Beginnings
	Echo	ultrasonic waves
	Electro	electricity
		Endings
About tests and procedures	Ectomy	removal of
	Gram	picture
	graph or graphy	process of taking a picture
	Otomy	making a cut in/removing a part of
	Scopy	use of instrument for viewing
	Stomy	create an opening in
	Plasty	modifying the shape of/repairing

Some of commonly used endings about specialists and specialties:

Purpose	Ending Words	Description
About specialties and specialists	Ology	study of a part of the body
	ologist	a specialist working for a specific part of the body or a specific disease
	iatry	medical treatment
	Iatrist	a specialist providing specific treatment

Chapter 3:

Root Words

Be Familiar with Root Words as Well

Usually, the root of a medical term is a body part. Using the example described in the previous chapter, cardio is the root of echocardiogram. It means heart. Here are some most commonly used word roots from the medical vocabulary:

Body Part	Root Word	Group
veins and arteries	vas or vasc	Cardiovascular system
blood	hem or hemo or sangu	
blood vessels	angi or angio	
veins	ven or veno or phleb or phlebo	
aorta	Aort	
arteries	arteri or arterio	

Medical Terminology

brain	Enceph/ Ceph	parts of the head
nose	Rhino	
eardrum	tympan or myringo	
tooth	odont or dento	
skull	Crani	
eye	ophthalm or oculo	
ear	Oto	
tongue	Lingu	
liver	hepat or hepato	organs in the digestive system
gallbladder	Cholecyst	
esophagus	esoph or esopha	
large intestine	Colo	
stomach	gastr or gastro	
small intestine	Ileo/duodeno/jejuno	
muscles	Myo	muscles and bones
shoulder	Scapula	
arm	brachi or brachio	
wrist	carp or carpo	
rib	cost or costo	
back	Dorsa	
bones	oste or osteo	
foot	pod or podo or ped or pedo	

chest	thorac or thoraco	
lung	pneumo or pleura	
breast	mamm or mammo	rest of the body
blood clot	thromb or thrombo	
kidney	Neph	

Tip: Group them into body parts, so it's easier to remember.

Combine Beginnings, Roots, and Endings

Now let's see how to put those beginnings, roots, and endings together. Use the tables above as guides. Let's use the word cardio as an example.

Cardi		itis
Root		Ending
body part: heart		medical problem: inflammation

Cardi + itis = inflammation of the heart

Cardi		Ology
Root		Ending
body part: heart		specialty: study of a part of the body

Cardi + ology = study of the heart

Cardio		Myo		pathy
beginning		Root		ending
body part: heart		body part: muscles		medical problem: disease

Cardio + myo + pathy = disease of the heart muscle

Medical Terminology

Echo	Cardio	graphy
Beginning	Root	ending
test and procedure: ultrasonic waves	body part: heart	test and procedure: process of making a picture

Echo + cardio + graphy = taking a picture of the heart using ultrasonic waves

Another example is the word colo or colon.

Colo		ostomy
Root		ending
body part: colon		test and procedure: opening of

Colo + stomy = creating an opening in the colon.

Colo		itis
Root		ending
body part: colon		medical problem: inflammation

Colo + itis = inflammation of the colon

Colo		ectomy
Root		Ending
body part: colon		test and procedure: removal of

Colo + ectomy = removal of the colon

Going back to the first example, Transesophageal Echocardiogram, let's divide the words per set.

Set 1: Transesophageal

Trans	eshophag	eal
Beginning	Root	ending
direction: across	body part: esophagus	Meaning: pertaining to

Trans + esophag + eal = going across the esophagus

Set 2: Echocardiogram

Echo	cardio	gram
Beginning	root	ending
test and procedure: ultrasonic waves	body part: heart	test and procedure: picture recording

Echo + cardio + gram = recording a picture of the heart using ultrasonic waves

Therefore, Transesophageal + Echocardiogram = a procedure where a patient swallows a tube that goes across the esophagus to record a picture of the heart using ultrasonic waves.

It also helps to know whether the root word refers to an internal or an external part of the body.

External Root Words

In the following table, you'll find the most common root words concerning the **outer** part of the body and its functions.

Exterior Root Word	What it Pertains to	Example	Meaning
Acr/ Acro	the extremities	**Acro**meg-aly	abnormally large upper and lower extremities (hands, feet, etc.) brought about by an increased production of growth hormone
Axill/ Axillo	the armpits	**Axill**ary	pertaining to the axilla Hence, **Axill**ary lymphade-nopathy is the enlargement of diseased lymph nodes in the axilla characterized by swollen armpits.
Blephar/ Blepharo	the eyelid	**Blepha-ro**plasty	the surgical repair of the eyelid
Brachi/ Brachio	the arm	**Brachi**al-gia	severe pain in the arm
Bucc/ Bucco	the cheek	**Bucc**al	means anything relating to the cheek Hence, Buccal mucosa refers to the interior lining of the cheek.
Canth/ Cantho	angle of the eyelids	**Canth**ot-omy	minor procedure where incision of tissues at the angle of the eye is performed to reduce pressure in orbital compart-ment syndrome, or to gain access to the bony orbit.

Capit/ Capito	the head/ shaped like a head	**Capit**ate bone	the largest hand bone at the center of the wrist that is shaped like a rounded head.
Carp/ Carpo	the wrist	**Carpo**p-tosis	a condition characterized by paralyzed extensor muscles of the hand and the fingers
Caud/ Caudo	the hind part/ tail/ down-ward	**Caud**al anesthe-sia	anesthesia performed by inject-ing a local anesthetic agent into the lower end of the sacrum and coccyx (tail bone) This provides pain relief from the umbilical (navel) region and below.
Cephal/ Cephalo	the head	**Cephalo**-hemato-ma	Occurring in infants, it pertains to a traumatic, solidified clot-ting of blood that takes place beneath the inner skin of the newborn's head. It does not affect the brain cells, but it does bring about a pooling of blood from the injured blood vessels, which lie between the baby's skull and the internal layers of the skin.
Cervic/ Cervico	the neck, such as of the body, or of the uterus (which is also called cervix)	**Cervi**-**co**genic headache	refers to a secondary headache brought about by a lesion or an injury in the neck (cervical spine)

Prefix	Meaning	Term	Definition
Cheil/ Cheilo/ Chil/ Chilo	the lips	**Cheilo**sis	inflamed lip corners, accompanied by redness, scaling, and cracking of the mouth corners This may be caused by Candida infection, or vitamin deficiencies.
Cheir/ Cheiro/ Chir/ Chiro	the hand	**Cheiro-pompho-lyx**	severely itchy skin eruptions on the sides of the fingers and the palms, made up of small blisters
Cili/ Cilio	eyelid, eyelash, relating to the eyelid or the eyelash	**Ciliary muscle**	a smooth muscle ring situated in the middle layer of the eye It regulates accommodation for viewing things at different distances. It is also responsible for controlling the flow of the aqueous humor
Derm/ Derma/ Dermato/ Dermo	the skin	**Derma-titis**	inflammation of the skin, caused by allergy
Dors/ Dorsi/ Dorso	back part/ posterior	**Dorsiflex-ion**	the backward bending of the foot or the hand
Faci/ Facio	the face	**Facios-capulo-humeral Muscular Dystro-phy**	is a rare inherited disorder, which begins by affecting the skeletal muscles of the face It then proceeds to affect the shoulders (scapula), and the upper arms (humeral). It involves the progressive weakening of the skeletal muscles in these areas.

Gingiv/ Gingivo	the gums	**Gingiv**itis	Inflammation of the gums
Gloss/ Glosso	the tongue	**Gloss**ody-nia	pain in the tongue, characterized by a burning sensation
Gnath/ Gnatho	the jaws	Orthog-**nath**ic	pertains to maintaining jaws in their correct relation and dimension. An Orthognathic surgery means an operation conducted to fix jaw deformities due to size or position. .
Inguin/ Inguino	the groin	**Inguino**-dynia	Post-surgical pain felt after the operation of an **inguin**al hernia An **Inguin**al hernia occurs when the tissues of the intestines push through the base of the abdomen. It appears as a lump in the groin. It also reveals itself as an enlargement of the scrotum in males.
Irid/ Irido	the iris of the eye	**Irido**ci-clitis	inflammation of the iris as well as the ciliary parts of the eye
Labi/ Labio	lips/ lip-like	**Labi**a	the lip-like skin folds of the vulva which serves as a protection to the opening of the vagina.
Lapar/ Laparo	the abdomen	**Laparo**s-copy	a surgical operation where a fiber-optic gadget is introduced via the abdominal wall, to allow the surgeon to see the organs within the abdomen This is often done to for diagnosis of abdominal diseases, or as part of a surgical procedure within the abdomen.

Later/ Latero	the side/ parts of the body which are farthest from the middle	Bilateral, Unilateral	means on both sides Hence, Bi**later**al micromastia refers to the underdevelopment of tissues in both breasts after puberty. In the same way, uni**later**al hearing loss refers to single-sided deafness, where only one ear is affected.
Lingu/ Lingo/ Linguo	the tongue	**Lin-guo**gingi-val	pertains to the tongue and the gums Hence, a **linguo**gingival groove during the embryonic stage refers to the furrow which separates the mandibular part of the tongue from the rest of the mandible.
Mamm/ Mamma/ Mammo	breasts	**Mammo**-gram	is an x-ray examination of the breasts
Mast/ Masto	breast	Gyneco-**mast**ia	the abnormal enlargement of breasts in males due to hormonal imbalances This is a possible side effect of hormone replacement therapy.
Nas/ Naso	the nose	**Naso**ga-stric	pertains to the mouth and the stomach (gastric) Hence, a **Naso**gastric intubation is a medical procedure where a plastic tube (**naso**gastric tube) is introduced via the nose, through the throat, and into the stomach, for assisted ventilation.

Occipit/ Occipito	the back of the head	Occipital bone	refers to a saucer-shaped bone located at the lower back area of the skull It contains the back portion of the brain.
Ocul/ Oculo	the eye	Oculogy-ric	pertains to the elevation of the visual gaze in both eyes An oculogyric crisis is an untoward reaction to medical disorders or pharmaceuticals which is manifested by a lengthy, uncontrollable, upward deviation of the person's eyes.
Odont/ Odonto	the teeth	Odonto-ma	a benign tumor associated with the development of the teeth It is brought about by the abnormal growth of normal dental tissue.
Omphal/ Omphalo	the umbi-licus	Ompha-loma	is a tumor situated in the umbilicus
Onych/ onycho	the nails	Parony-chia	painful and pus-filled soft tissue infection involving the finger-nails The chronic type of paronychia is usually caused by a fungal infection (Candidiasis).
Opthalm/ Opthlamo	the eyes	Opthal-moscopy	a non-invasive medical procedure where the eye doctor (ophthalmologist) utilizes an opthalmoscope to view and check the inside of the eye

Optic/ Optico/ Opto	sight	**Optom**-etry	An assessment method done to evaluate vision and to determine whether glasses or contacts are required to fix a visual problem
Or/ Oro	the mouth	**Oro**pha-ryngeal	Involves the mouth as well as the pharynx Hence, **Oro**pharyngeal dysphagia pertains to difficulty in swallowing due to abnormalities or malfunction not just in the throat but also in the mouth.
Ot/ Oto	the ear/s	**Ot**itis media	Inflammation of the middle ear brought about by an infection (caused by either bacteria or a virus) spreading to the Eustachian tube
Papill/ Papillo	the nipple	**Papillo**-ma	a non-cancerous tumor in the breast ducts which consists of mammary epithelium (cells which make up the breast's duct wall linings) They block the duct fully and have fronds that resemble fingers.
Pelv/ Pelvo	pelvis	**Pelv**iec-tasis	the dilation of the renal pelvis
Phall/ Phallo	the penis	**Phal**-loplasty	a surgical procedure performed to augment or to repair the penis
Pil/ Pilo	hair	**Pilo**cystic	term used to denote a cyst which contains hair

Pod/ Podo	the foot/ feet	**Pod**iatry	a branch of medicine which is dedicated to the treatment, both medical and surgical, of the foot and other parts of the lower extremities
Rhin/ Rhino	the nose	**Rhino**r- rhea	pertains to a condition where the nasal cavity is persistently filled with substantial amounts of mucous fluid
Somat/ Somato	body	**Somato**- genic	relates to the body Hence, **Somato**genic diseases refer to illnesses which origi- nate from the parts of the body. These are the opposite of **psy- cho**genic diseases wherein the cause of the illness is of mental origin.
Steth/ Stetho	the chest	**Stetho**- scope	an acoustic tool, usually placed against the chest, used for listening to the inner sounds of the body, so as to aid in diagnosis.
Stomat/ Stomato	mouth/ opening	**Stoma**- titis	inflamed mucus membranes of the mouth
Tal/ Talo	the ankle	Sub**tal**ar disloca- tion	the dislocation of a bone in the hindfoot, which connects with the tibia (shinbone) and the fibula (lateral leg bone)
Tars/ Tarso	foot	**Tars**algia	pain experienced in the rear area of the foot This commonly occurs in indi- viduals with flat feet.

Thorac/ Thoraco	the chest/ thorax	Thora- centesis	a sterile procedure wherein fluid is removed from the pleural space (the space between the two pleural membranes of the lung) This is done through the insertion of a needle via the chest wall.
Tracheo/ Trachelo	the neck/ neckline	Trachelo- myitis	inflammation of the neck muscles
Trich/ Tricho	hair/ like hair	Trichiasis	a condition where the direction of the growth of the eyelash is changed The lashes end up growing inward to the direction of the eyeball. Consequently, the hairs may rub against the eye and can cause irritation and even corneal damage.
Ventr/ Ventri/ Ventro	the front part of the body	Ventro- gluteal IM	a deep muscular injection into the gluteus medius on the outer surface of the pelvis

Internal Root Words

In the following table, you'll find the most common root words pertaining to the *inner* parts of the body and their functions.

Internal Root Word	What it Pertains to	Example	Meaning
Acanth/ Acantho	spinous/ with spikes	**Acantho**-cyte	a red blood cell with a spinous cell membrane
Aer/ Aero	Gas	**Aero**sinus-itis	inflamed nasal sinuses, more commonly experienced by deep sea divers and high altitude flyers This is caused by the difference between internal sinus cavity pressure and the atmospheric pressure.
Alge/ Algo/ Algio	pain	An**alge**sics	a group of pharmaceutical drugs used to obtain relief from pain
Andro	masculine	**Andro**blas-toma	tumor in the testicles
Bronch/ Bronchi/ Broncho	the bronchus (part of the respiratory system that directs air into the lungs)	**Broncho**c-onstrictor	an element or a drug which causes the airways in the lungs to constrict and narrow It can potentially trigger an asthma attack.
Bronchiol/ Bronchio	bronchiole/s (smaller airways which branch off the bronchi)	**Bronchi**-olitis	a severe viral infection affecting the lungs where there is inflammation of the bronchioles This occurs more commonly in infants and younger kids. The common causative agent is the respiratory syncytial virus.

Carcin/ Carcino	cancer	**Carcino**gen	any substance, usually a chemical, which is capable of causing cancer When these come in contact with the body in harmful amounts, **carcino**genesis occurs. The latter refers to the development of cancer.
Cardi/ Cardio	the heart	**Cardio**my-opathy	any clinical condition which affects the muscles of the heart and causes diminishing of the force of cardiac contraction This effect reduces the cardiac output and effi-ciency of blood circula-tion.
Cellul/ Cellulo	cell	**Cellul**itis	an infection in the skin and in the underlying tis-sues caused by bacteria, often by streptococci, which gains access to the skin through a wound
Cerebell/ Cerebello	cerebellum	**Cerebell**ar ataxia	refers to the irregular, spasmodic, and involun-tary movements brought about by diseases of the cerebellum or an injury to the cerebellum
Cerebr/ Cerberi/ Cerbero	cerebrum	**Cerebro**-vascular disease	any medical condition which affects the arteries within the brain or the arteries supplying blood to the brain

Chol/ Chole	bile	**Chol**angiography	a diagnostic procedure where a contrast medium is used to render the bile ducts visible through an X-ray It is done to check for the presence of biliary stones or tumors, or to determine if there is narrowing of the bile ducts.
Cholecyst/ Cholecysto	the gallbladder	**Cholecyst**ectomy	the removal of the gallbladder through surgical means
Chrom/ Chromo	color	**Chrom**atogenous	producing color
Col/ Colo	colon	**Colo**stomy	a surgical procedure wherein part of the colon is taken out via an incision made in the wall of the abdomen An artificial opening is then made in this colon segment, which serves as an exit point of feces. The fecal matter will be eliminated into a bag affixed to the patient's skin.
Colp/ Colpo	the vagina	**Colpo**scopy	A diagnostic procedure where the cervix and the vagina are visually inspected through a magnifying device (**Colp**oscope) This is done as part of a screening procedure for cancer.

Cost/ Costo	rib	**Cost**algia	pain in the chest area caused by injury to one of the ribs
Cry/ Cryo	cold	**Cryo**sur-gery	a therapeutic procedure, where extremely low tem-peratures are utilized for the destruction of tissues

Alternatively, the cold may be used to promote adhesion between a tool and the tissue. |
| **Crypt/ Crypto** | hidden | **Crypt**orchi-dism | a developmental disorder in newborn boys, charac-terized by failure of the testes to drop into the scrotum |
| **Cutane/ Cutaneo** | skin | Sub**cutane**-ous | The area underneath the skin; for example, a subcutaneous injection is given just below the skin. |
| **Cyan/ Cyano** | blue | **Cyano**sis | a skin discoloration, where the extremities of the face turn bluish, as a result of excessive amounts of deoxygenated hemoglobin in the blood

Cyanosis of the lips is indicative of heart failure or chronic obstructive pulmonary disease. |

Cysti/ Cyst/ Cysto	cyst	**Cyst**icer-cosis	a severe albeit rare condition, where there is an infestation of parasitic cysts within the muscles and even in the brain This is brought about by the infestation of pork tapeworm.
Cyt/ Cyto	cell	**Cyto**logy	pertains to the study of individual cells It is useful in medicine particularly when it comes to detecting anomalous, possibly malignant cells in cancer screening.
Dipl/ Diplo	double	**Dipl**opia	clinical term for double vision
Duoden/ Duodeno	duodenum	**Duoden**itis	inflamed duodenum, which creates ambiguous gastrointestinal symp-toms
Encephal/ Encephalo	brain	Electro**en-cephalo**-gram	a diagnostic procedure done to check for abnor-malities in the brain's electrical activity It is done by tracking and recording brain wave patterns.
Enter/ Entro	intestine	Gastro-**enter**itis	infection of the stomach and the intestines, usually due to a viral or bacterial causative agent

| Episi/Epi-sio | the vulva | Episiorrha-phy | surgical repair of a laceration of the vulva

This usually is done after an **episio**tomy where the perineum and the posterior vaginal wall are cut by the obstetrician during the second phase of labor.

Episiotomy is performed to ease the passage of the infant through a bigger opening, and to prevent irregular tearing of the vulva. |
|---|---|---|---|
| **Eryth/ Erythro** | red | **Eryth**ro-cytes | red blood cells |
| **Esophag/ Esophago** | esophagus | **Esophag**itis | inflammation of the esophageal lining |
| **Fibr/ Fibro** | fibers | **Fibro**sis | scar tissue overgrowth, caused by the body's exaggerated healing mechanism as a response to an infection, a wound, or inflammation

For instance, in the case of esophagitis, the thick scar tissue ends up narrowing the esophagus and causing difficulty in swallowing. |

Galact/ Galacto	milk	**Galactor**-rhea	excessive production of milk or milk-like discharge from the nipples It can happen to non-pregnant women, menopausal women, men, and even babies. This is often the result of high levels of prolactin, a hormone that triggers the production of milk.
Gastr/ Gastro	stomach	**Gastro**sto-my	a surgical procedure where an opening is created in the stomach, so that a feeding tube may be attached
Glyc/ Glyco	sugar	**Glyco**penia	sugar deficiency
Gynec/ Gyneco	female	**Gyneco**logy	a medical practice which specifically deals with female reproductive health
Hemat/ Hemato	blood	**Hemat**oma	localized pooling of blood ,(often solidified) brought about by bleeding from a vessel that has ruptured
Hepat/ Hepato/ Hepatic	the liver	**Hepato**-megaly	enlargement of the liver
Heter/ Hetero	dissimilar	**Hetero**ch-romia	a congenital condition where there is a difference in the color of the skin, the hair, but most often in the iris. (eg. one eye is brown and the other is blue) However, it can also be the effect of a medical condition or an injury.

Medical Terminology

Hidr/ Hidro	sweat	Hyper**hi-dro**sis	excessive sweating
Hist/ His-to/ Histio	tissue	**Histo**logy	refers to the study of tissues, as well as their cellular structures and function This field is valuable to medicine particularly in the diagnosis of illnesses.
Hom/ Homo/ Home/ Homeo	similar	**Homeo**plasia	the development of new, similar tissue
Hydr/ Hydro	water	**Hydro**cele	a condition where the space around the testes is filled with fluid This causes tender swelling in the scrotum and may be brought about by an injury sustained by the testes, by inflammation, or by tumors.
Hyster/ Hystero	the uterus	**Hyster**ectomy	the operative removal of the uterus for a therapeutic cause

Iatr/ Iatro	treatment	**Iatro**genic	suggests a link to treatment Thus, an **Iatro**genic anemia (low hemoglobin and hematocrit values) is the result of the recurrent removal of large volumes of blood. This could be because of repeated laboratory testing for diagnostic or monitoring purpose, or surgical blood loss. In such cases, the cure becomes the cause.
Jejun/ Jejuno	jejunum (mid-part of the small intestine)	**Jejuno**stomy	a surgical procedure where an opening is created through the wall of the jejunum, so that a plastic tube may be inserted for feeding
Kerat/Kerato	the eye's cornea	**Kerato**malacia	a disease of the eyes brought about a by lack of vitamin A In this condition, the cornea becomes cloudy and ulcerated and eventually, perforated. This could lead to loss of vision.
Laryng/ Laryngo	the larynx	**Laryng**itis	inflamed larynx

Leuk/ Leuko	white	**Leuk**emia	the excessive propagation of immature white blood cells, which leads to the incompetence of vital body organs such as the spleen, the brain, and the liver, once the abnormal cells infiltrate them
Lip/ Lipo/ Lipid/ Lipido	fat	**Lipo**sarco-ma	an unusual type of connective tissue cancer, where the abnormal cells look like fat cells Swelling is experienced in the thighs and in the abdominal region.
Lith/ Litho	stone (usually in the kidney or the gall-bladder)	**Litho**tomy	surgical removal of stones from areas of the urinary tract
Lymph/ Lympho	the lymph vessels	**Lymph**an-giography	a diagnostic test conduct-ed through the injection of a contrast agent into the lymph vessels, in order to make any abnor-malities visible through X-rays
Melan/ Melano	black	**Melano**-cytes	cells that form melanin
Men/ Meno	menstrua-tion	**Men**orrha-gia	abnormally disproportion-ate menstrual bleeding

Mening/ Meningo	meninges	**Mening**itis	inflamed and infected meninges, with a bacteria or a virus as the causative agent

This fatal condition is accompanied by severe headaches, photosensitivity, and stiffening of the muscles. |
| **Metr/ Metra/ Metro** | uterus | **Metr**orrhagia | irregular bleeding from the uterus that is experienced between the woman's monthly periods |
| **My/ Myo** | muscle | **My**algia | clinical term for muscular pain |
| **Myel/ Myelo** | the spine or the bone marrow | **Myelo**sclerosis | proliferation of fibrous tissue in the bone marrow

This impairs the bone marrow's competence in producing blood cells. |
| **Myring/ Myringo** | the eardrum | **Myringo**plasty | a corrective operative procedure where a hole in the eardrum is closed through tissue grafting |
| **Nat/ Nato** | birth | Neo**nate** | a newborn baby, less than four months |
| **Necr/ Necro** | death | **Necr**osis | refers to the death of tissue cells, when the supply of blood is not sufficient (ischemia), or as a result of an infection (such as in the case of tuberculosis)

It can also be caused by damage brought about by extreme temperatures, or exposure to radiation or harmful chemicals. |

Medical Terminology

Nephr/ Nephro	the kidney/s	**Nephro**cal-cinosis	the presence of calcium deposits in one or both kidneys
Oophor/ Oophoro	the ovaries	**Oophor**ec-tomy	surgical removal of the ovaries, as a last resort treatment for ovarian cysts or ovarian cancer
Orchi/ Orchid/ Orchido/ Orchio	the testes	**Orchi**tis	inflamed testes accompanied by high temperature, severe pain, and swelling around the area When this occurs post-puberty, it is commonly due to the mumps virus.
Oss/ Os-seo/ Ossi/ Ost/ Osteo	the bones	**Osteo**my-elitis	an infection, usually of bacterial origin, of the bone and in the bone marrow
Palat/ Palato	the palate (roof of the mouth)	**Palato-**plasty	surgical reconstruction of a cleft palate
Path/ Patho	disease	**Patho**gen	causative agent of a disease, usually a microorganism
Periton/ Peritone	the peritoneum	**Periton**itis	inflamed peritoneum This is usually brought about by entry of bacteria and digestive fluids into the abdominal cavity, through a punctured stomach or intestinal wall.
Pharmac/ Pharmaco	drugs	**Pharmaco-**dynamics	the term which pertains to the way the body reacts to, synthesizes, and benefits from a pharmaceutical substance

Pharyng/ Pharyngo	the pharynx	**Pharyng**itis	inflamed pharynx usually due to a viral or bacterial pathogen It can also be caused by irritants such as smoking, foreign objects, and ingested corrosive substances.
Phleb/ Phlebo	vein	**Phleb**itis	the inflammation of a vein; usually occurs after injection of an irritant drug into the vein.
Phren/ Phreno	diaphragm	**Phren**ic nerve	a nerve which supplies the diaphragm It is essential for breathing. When injured or removed, half of the diaphragm will be rendered paralyzed.
Pleur/ Pleuro	the pleura	**Pleur**isy	inflamed pleura (membranes which envelop the lungs) due to infections of the lung, pulmonary embolism, or cancer of the lung
Pneum/ Pneuma/ Pneumo/ Pneumato	the lungs	**Pneumo-**thorax	a potentially fatal condition where air leaks into the pleural cavity (the gaps between the two pleura surrounding the lungs) This will eventually lead to lung collapse, because of pleural compression on the lungs.

Poli/ Polio	gray	**Polio**my-elitis	an infectious condition caused by a viral patho-gen The severe type tends to affect the brain (especially the nervous system's gray matter) and the spinal cord. When this happens, the disease becomes fatal.
Proct/ Procto	the anus or the rectum	**Proct**itis	inflamed rectum com-monly accompanied by pain, bleeding, and pus. It occurs in conditions such as Crohn's disease and ulcerative colitis. It may also be caused by gonorrhea and other sexually transmitted infections.
Pulmon/ Pulmono	the lungs	**Pulmon**ary hyperten-sion	a condition wherein there is an abnormally elevated blood pressure in the arteries which provide blood to the lungs
Pyel/ Pyelo	the pelvis/ the kidneys	**Pyel**one-phritis	inflamed kidney/s often due to a bacterial caus-ative agent
Rect/ Recto	the rectum	**Recto**cele	a condition wherein the tissues of the vaginal wall are weakened and the back wall of the vagina bulges inward and down-ward because the rectum is pushing against it

Sacr/ Sacro	the sacrum	**Sacr**algia	this is the pain experienced in the sacrum, usually associated with disc prolapse This is due to the pressure created on the spinal nerve.
Salping/ Salpingo	the fallopian tube	**Salping**itis	inflamed fallopian tube/s, which may be due to a pelvic inflammatory disease but is more often brought about by sexually transmitted infections
Sarc/ Sarco	flesh	**Sarco**idosis	a sporadic inflammatory disease of unknown origin which affects tissues around the body, most frequently the skin, the liver, and the lymph nodes
Sept/ Septo	contamination	**Sept**icemia	a deadly condition where there is fast propagation of bacteria which release toxins into the bloodstream This happens when the pathogen escapes from the local area of infection (eg. an abscess). This commonly affects individuals with poor immune systems, such as cancer patients, HIV patients, or those taking medications which suppress the immune system.
Splen/ Spleno	the spleen	Hyper-**splen**ism	an overly active spleen

Spondyl/ Spondylo	the verte-bra	**Spondy-lo**sis	a spinal disorder in which the arch of the 5th lumbar vertebra is not made up of normal bone as it should be, but is instead composed of soft, fibrous tissue which is weak and susceptible to damage
Ten/ Tend/ Tendo/ Teno	tendon	**Tend**initis	inflamed tendon, frequently due to an injury or excessive use
Testicul/ Testiculo	testis	**Testicul**ar Femini-zation Syndrome	(now more commonly referred to as Complete Androgen Insensitivity Syndrome) In this case, the infants are born as girls with vaginal pouches sans uterus or any other female reproductive organs. A testes is present in the abdomen or in the inguinal region. However, the body's tissues are unable to respond to testosterone which is responsible for the development of male sexual characteristics.
Therm/ Thermo	heat	**Thermog-**raphy	a method where the temperature patterns of the skin's surface are documented as images
Thyr/ Thyro	the thyroid gland	Hypo**thy-ro**idism	a condition where the thyroid hormone production in the body is less than normal

Tonsill/ Tonsillo	the tonsils	**Tonsill**ec-tomy	a surgical operation conducted for removal of the tonsils
Trache/ Tracheo	the trachea	**Trache**os-tomy	an emergency procedure, done by creating an opening in the windpipe when the person's upper airway is obstructed This way, a tube, sometimes connected to an oxygen supply or ventilator, can be inserted.
Tympan/ Tympano	the ear-drum	**Tympan**os-tomy tube	a tube which is introduced into the eardrum, to avoid fluid buildup in the middle ear
Ur/ Ure/ Urea/ Ureo/ Urin/ Uri-no/ Uro	urine	**Urin**alysis	a diagnostic test conducted to measure the urine's physical characteristics, such as the color and the concentration
Urethr/ Urethero	urethra	**Urethro**-cele	a female deformity wherein the tissues in the vagina's front wall are weakened, thus allowing the urethra to bulge back and down into the vagina
Vesic/ Vesi-co	the bladder	**Vesico**uret-eral reflux	the retrograde flow of urine from the bladder back to the kidneys In normal situations, the flow is from the kidney, through the ureters, and toward the bladder.
Viscer/ Viscero	internal organs (the viscera)	**Viscero**pto-sis	the prolapse/ downward displacement of the internal organs within the abdomen

Xanth/ Xantho	yellow	Xan-thochromia	yellowish discoloration, which is indicative of the presence of bilirubin in the cerebrospinal fluid
Xer/ Xero	dry	Xerophthla-mia	dryness of the eyes, involving the cornea and the conjunctiva, caused by lack of vitamin A

Directional Root Words

The following are the most common directional terms that are encountered in medicine. In medical terminology, you'll notice that they're often joined together or affixed to another word (e.g. a body part), in order to denote a specific route. Every day, in the medical setting, they are used to specify an intravenous site, the particular location of an infection or an injury, or the direction towards which a patient must be moved.

> » **Anterior** or **Ventral** means the front of the body or toward the front part of the human anatomy.

Hence, the **ante**cubital vein refers to a vein situated in the front part of the body, specifically in front of the elbow.

> » **Posterior** and **Dorsal** are the opposite of ventral, since they refer to the rear part of the body or the direction toward the back of the human anatomy.

For instance, the **dorso**gluteal injection site is located in the buttocks, specifically in the upper outer quadrant of the gluteal muscles. An experienced medical practitioner finds it easy by dividing the cheek of the buttocks into four corresponding quadrants and then inserting the needle into the superior lateral region.

> » **Superior** or **Cranial** means upper. It pertains to a position which is situated higher than or above a body part.

A surgically created connection between the flesh and the bladder is required for draining the urine of patients suffering from urinary tract obstructions. Therefore, a **supra**pubic catheter is inserted to the bladder via a skin incision made slightly *above* the pubic bone.

» As mentioned previously, **Caudal** means tail. A synonymous directional word is **Inferior**. As a directional term, both mean lower. They pertain to a position which is situated lower than or below a body part.

The **inferior** vena cava, for instance, is a major vein which transports deoxygenated blood coming from the lower part of your body toward your heart's right atrium.

Likewise, when a doctor performs a cephalo**caudal** assessment, this means s/he assesses the patient from head to toe.

» As stated previously, Lateral means at the side or toward the side of the body. **Latero**collis, therefore, is the involuntary movement of the head from side to side. This is observed in patients with neck dystonia. Fittingly, **Antero**colis pertains to the abnormal forward movement of the head.

» Whereas lateral is used to describe a direction *away* from the middle of the body, the term **Medial** means the opposite. It pertains to the middle or going toward the center of the human anatomy.

If a patient is experiencing antero**medial** knee pain, then the front and center part of his knee is in pain.

» **Proximal**, when used to describe a limb, refers to the part which is nearest to the torso or to the joint.

» Conversely, **Distal** is used to refer to the site which is farthest from the torso or the joint.

When a pediatrician says that a child manifests normal **Proximo**distal development, he means to say that the motor skills in body parts which are closest to the torso develop earlier than the motor skills in body parts which are further (distal) from the trunk. In other words, the child will first learn how to wave his arms before learning how to paint pictures with his fingers.

» **Superficial** is used to refer to a position which is closest to the body's surface.

» On the other hand, **Deep** pertains to a position which is distant or away from the body's surface.

Example: The body's fascia serve as protective paddings. They work to decrease the fiction of muscular force.

The **Superficial** fascia makes up the layer below the skin.

However, the **Deep** fascia is found further within the body since it envelops the blood vessels, the nerves, and the bones.

Ready for a word-building activity now?

Word Building Exercise

Part 1 - Instruction: Choose the correct word part to *fill in the blanks*.

1.   Define: Inflammation of the throat. **Answer:** _____

[fill in the blank]-itis

- ot
- tonsill
- encephal
- rhin
- neur
- laryng

2.   Define: Specialist working with the nerves. **Answer:** _____

[fill in the blank]-ologist

- cardi
- ophthal
- neur
- gastr
- mamm
- colon

3.   Define: the study of the bones. **Answer:** _____

[fill in the blank]-ology

- odont
- rhin
- phleb
- ot
- cardi
- oste

4.   Define: a slow heartbeat. **Answer:** _____

brady-[fill in the blank]

- derma
- gastro
- rhino
- lacrima
- cardia
- oculo

5.   Define: inflammation of the brain. **Answer:** _____

[fill in the blank]-itis

- ot
- hepa
- gastr
- encephal
- tonsill
- col

6.   Define: inflammation of the area around the heart. **Answer:** _____

[fill in the blank]-card-[fill in the blank]

- chloro
- itis
- micro
- endo
- oscopy
- peri

7.   Define: Disease of the nerves. **Answer:** _____

neuro-[fill in the blank]

- megaly
- scopy
- logy
- itis
- gram
- pathy

8.   Define: A picture taken of the heart using electricity. **Answer:** _____

[fill in the blank]-cardio-[fill in the blank]

- hyper
- gram
- ologist
- echo
- scope
- electro

9. Define: too much cholesterol in the blood. **Answer:** _____

[fill in the blank]-cholesterol-[fill in the blank]

- pathy
- itis
- exo
- hyper
- megalo
- emia

10. Define: Inflammation of the nose. **Answer:** _____

[fill in the blank]-itis

- gastro
- ot
- laryng
- neph
- hepat
- rhin

Part 2 – Instruction: Choose the correct answer to the following questions:

11. What body system does osteoporosis affect? **Answer:** _____
- heart
- bone
- eye

12. Which word does not belong? **Answer:** _____
- hypersensitivity
- hyperactivity
- hypotension

13. Is Hepatitis inflammation of the liver? **Answer:** _____
- true
- false

14. Is Pericarditis inflammation of the kidney? **Answer:** _____
- true
- false

15. If a doctor wants to look at the colon of a patient, what is this procedure called? **Answer:** _____

   - Microscopy
   - Mammography
   - Colonoscopy

Great job! Correct answers are in chapter 11.

Chapter 4:

Pronouncing Medical Terms

Majority of medical terms are challenging to pronounce. In some cases, a letter might be pronounced differently in two ways. In others meanwhile, some letters are pronounced silently. Rules of pronunciation are not the same for every letter and word. However, learning the basic and most commonly used rules can help medical and non-medical people to pronounce similar medical terms. Featured here are some of the most commonly used medical terms and how to pronounce them.

A. Sounds in Pronunciation

1. Beginning with "j", pronounced as: "j"
   Example: **j**aundice

2. Beginning with "sk", pronounced as: "sk"
   Example: **sk**eletal

3. Beginning with "gy", pronounced as: "guy"
   Example: **gy**necologist

4. Beginning with "cho", pronounced as: "k"
   Example: **ch**olesterol

5. Beginning with "ce" or "ci", pronounced as: "si"
   Example: **ce**liac

6. Beginning with "gi" or "ge", pronounced as: "j"
   Example: **gi**ardisis

7. Beginning with "kn", pronounced as: "n"
   Example: **kn**ock **kn**ees

8. Beginning with "cu" or "ca", pronounced as: "k"
    Example: **Cu**shing's syndrome

9. Beginning with "x", pronounced as: "z"
    Example: **x**erophthalmia

10. Beginning with "psy", pronounced as: "siy" with silent letter "p"
    Example: **psy**chology

11. Beginning with "n" and is followed by a vowel, pronounced as: "n"
    Example: **n**orovirus

12. Beginning with "ph", pronounced as: "f"
    Example: **ph**ysiotherapy

13. Beginning with "cy", pronounced as: "s"
    Conditions: if "cy" followed by "s", it is pronounced as "see"
    If "cy" followed by other letters, it is pronounced as "si"
    Example: **cy**toscopy, **cy**stocele vs. cytology

14. Beginning with "sch", pronounced as: "sk"
    Example: **sch**istosomiasis

15. Beginning with "pn", pronounced as: "n" with silent "p"
    Example: **pn**eumococcal

16. Beginning with "k" and is followed by a vowel, pronounced as: "k"
    Example: **k**idney

17. Beginning with "g" and is followed by a consonant, pronounced as:
    "guh"
    Example: **g**ranuloma

18. Beginning with "z", pronounced as: "z"
    Example: **z**ika virus

19. Beginning with "sc", pronounced as: "sk"
    Example: **sc**oliosis

20. Root word ending with "g", followed by "e" or "i", pronounced as:
    "j"
    Example: laryn**ge**al

21. Medical term with "oe" or "ae", pronounced as: "e"
    Example: oligomenorrh**oe**a

22. Beginning with "thy" or "ty", pronounced as: "thi" or "ti"
    Example: **thy**roid, **ty**phoid (except in typhus which is pronounced as "tee-foos")

23. Ending with "thy", pronounced as: pronounced as soft "thee"
    Example: trime**thy**laminuria

" For medical professionals, part of voicing their knowledge is to pronounce medical terms correctly. This ensures proper communication with other medical team members, providing successful medical care for patients.

B. Sound Exercise

Instruction: Choose the correct sound of the highlighted letters.

1. Laryn*ge*ctomy. **Answer:**_____
   - g
   - j
   - guh

2. *Gy*naecomastia. **Answer:** _____
   - guh
   - guy
   - juy

3. *Gi*ngivitis. **Answer:** _____
   - juh
   - chu
   - j

4. *Ph*imosis. **Answer:** _____
   - chi
   - p
   - f

5. *K*oilonychia. **Answer:** _____
   - ch
   - k
   - c

6. *Sc*leroderma. **Answer:** _____
   - sh
   - ch
   - sk

7. En*co*presis. **Answer:** _____
   - ch
   - k
   - s

8. Ty*ph*us. **Answer:** _____
   - s
   - ch
   - f

9. <u>Oe</u>sophageal. **Answer:** _____
    - a
    - o
    - e

10. <u>Neu</u>rone. **Answer:** _____
    - new
    - nu
    - ne

11. An<u>ae</u>mia. **Answer:** _____
    - o
    - a
    - e

12. Homo<u>cy</u>stinuria. **Answer:** _____
    - see
    - si
    - se

13. Masto<u>cy</u>tosis. **Answer:** _____
    - si
    - say
    - see

14. Ence<u>ph</u>alitis. **Answer:** _____
    - ch
    - f
    - s

15. Neuropa<u>thy</u>. **Answer:** _____
    - thee
    - thi
    - thy

Good job! Answers are in chapter 11.

Chapter 5:

Memorizing Medical Terms

Using different learning methods and tools can help memorizing medical terms easier. Given below are the most commonly used methods for memorizing medical terms quickly and easily:

A. Using Flashcards and Phone Apps

1. Word Flashcards

For visual learners, flashcards are a great option for memorizing. It allows learners to associate medical terms with visual cues, and helps them to connect and commit such terms to memory. It also provides a cheap alternative, especially to students who are always on a tight budget. Flashcards are cheap to make. They can be made at home using board paper and a pen or marker. They are the most inexpensive study aids that students can rely on.

Apart from being affordable, the process of making flashcards at home can help learners to rewrite medical terms repetitively. This can help them to remember medical terms more easily, thus making it easy to memorize words that they've learned.

For learners who are too busy to create flashcards at home, there are always ones that are available online, or in bookstores that are professionally made. What's more, pre-made flashcards often have images in them that can help learners to memorize medical terms visually.

2. Phone Apps

Another visual option is by using apps that are readily available on mobile devices and smart phones. By using phone apps, there is no need to carry books or flashcards all the time. This is a good option for learners who are always travelling.

Medical Terminology

There are many apps that can help learners to memorize medical terms, but only a few are reliable. Given below are a number of Android and iOS apps that are helpful in memorizing medical terms:

For Android Phones

»   App name: Med Term Scramble

Developer: Pearson Education

It is played like Scramble, but it uses only medical terms. It features more than 30 different lists or words. An iOS version is also available.

»   App name: Learn Medical Terminology

Developer: MedTerminologyForCare UK

This app features interactive e-learning courses and medical terms exercises. There are also lists of prefixes, roots and suffixes to discover – all for free.

»   App name: Medical Terminology Quiz

Developer: Quetzal Inc.

This app features a multiple choice quiz on twelve different topics discussing the anatomy of the human body.

»   App name: Medical Terms EN

Developer: Tech IndiaNa Pvt. Ltd.

This app features commonly used medical terms, including diseases, symptoms, and tests. It also has a voice-enabled search, word completion, and other smart options.

»   App name: Medical Terminologies

Developer: Medical Group Soft

This app is a simple, but comprehensive dictionary of medical terms. It also works when offline.

»   App name: Medical Terminology Flashcards

Developer: Simple Tree LLC

While it has pre-made flashcards, it also allows users to create their own cards. It features a progress tracker.

For iOS Phones

> » App name: Medical Terminology and Abbreviations

Developer: Air Capital Media LLC

It features a list of prefixes, abbreviations, and suffixes to help learners understand and memorize complicated medical words.

> » App name: Eponyms (for students)

Developer: Ossus GmbH

This app features a short description of medical eponyms including more than 1,700 common and complex medical terms.

> » App name: MCAT Flashcards – Kaplan National Practice Test

Developer: Kaplan

This app allows users to create flashcards choosing from 200 topics ranging from organic chemistry, general chemistry, physics, and biology.

> » App name: Taber's Medical Dictionary

Developer: Unbound Medicine, Inc.

This app features more than 65,000 medical terms with 1,200 photos. It also has 100+ videos and 32,000 audio.

> » App name: Med Term Scramble

Developer: Pearson Education

This app, also mentioned earlier, is available on Android phones as well.

> » App name: Psych Terms

Developer: Michael Quach

This app is a medical dictionary for terms related to psychiatry, psychology, and other mental health issues.

B. Using Visual Reminders

This applies not only when memorizing medical terms, but to all words as well. Using images to associate with words can help learners memorize terms effectively. Using images to represent medical terms can act as cues when trying to remember words. This works because the human brain is designed to save and remember images as information. For example, by saying the word baby, the mind visualizes an infant instead of spelling out the word itself.

C. Rewriting Medical Terms

With repetition, the memory process speeds up; that's why rewriting medical terms can improve memorization of those words, especially if done by hand. Typing words on a computer or a smart phone doesn't produce the same effect. Also, rewriting study notes can improve understanding of medical terms, making it easier to study them.

Tip: Writing medical terms and their definitions 5 to 10 times produces the best results.

Chapter 6:

Prefixes and Suffixes

Learning Prefix, Root, and Suffix

As mentioned, the easiest way to understand medical terms is to learn their parts: the beginning (prefix), middle (root), and ending (suffix). It is also the smartest way to memorize medical terms because almost all medical terms include all these three parts. Most importantly, almost all medical terms are based on a root word which is the core of a word, carrying its meaning.

1. Prefix – the Beginning

The prefix is a group of letters or a single letter, set before a word to change its meaning. For example, the word "unable" has a root word of able. When the prefix "un" is added, the meaning changes from being capable to being not capable. In the medical field, a prefix is a word added before a root word to provide additional information about the time involved, location of an organ, or number of parts.

2. Suffix – the Ending

The suffix is a group of letters or a single letter set after a word to also change its meaning. For example, the word "useful" has a root word of use. When "ful" was added at the end, its meaning became different. From being an act, it became as something that describes value. In the medical field, a suffix is a word added after a root word to include a procedure, disease, or condition.

3. Root Word – the Middle

The root word is sometimes in the middle or at the beginning of medical terms. The easiest way to memorize root words is by learning its Latin or Greek meaning. There is no need to learn long words as long as the root words are kept in mind. So, it's better to focus on root words instead. For a guide on basic medical root words, please refer to Chapter 2.

4. Word Combinations

Sometimes, medical terms may contain more than one root word. For example, there are 2 root words in the medical term "bronchogenic": "bronch" and "gen". The letter "o" was added to make pronunciation easier, while the suffix "ic" was added at the end.

Also, medical terms can be formed using a number of combinations:

prefix + root + suffix

root + suffix

prefix + root

Merely by learning prefixes, suffixes, and root words only, learners can already have vast knowledge of medical terms, making it easier to memorize such words.

The Most Important Prefixes

Given below is a table of the most indispensable prefixes in the medical field, accompanied by their meanings, and examples of their applications.

Pre-fix	Meaning	Example of the Meaning	Meaning of the Example
A	without, devoid of, not	**A**pnea	the absence of breathing
An	devoid of, without	**An**esthesia	without sensation

Alb	white	**Alb**inism	a condition where the affected individual has an abnormally white complexion, due to lack of melanin pigment in the skin as well as in the eyes and the hair
Auto	self	**Auto**lysis	a self-destructive mechanism of cells in which the cells are destroyed by their own enzymes
Bi	both, dual, twice	**Bi**cuspid	possessing dual cusps, which is seen in premolar teeth
Co/ Con/ Com	along with	**Con**genital heart disease	inborn defects which disrupt the normal mechanisms of the heart
De	down, to rid of	**De**pilatory	a chemical substance used for hair removal; typically used in cases of hirsutism (excessive and abnormal hair growth on the face and the body)
Dis	to rid of, to undo a natural state	**Dis**location	a joint injury wherein two or more of the bones are forcibly removed from their natural positions

Ex-tra/ Extro	external, beyond	**Extra**uterine pregnancy	the development of an embryo outside the uterus such as in an ectopic pregnancy
Hemi	half	**Hemi**plegia	when one half of the body is paralyzed
Hy-per	extreme, excessive, situated above	**Hyper**somno-lence	persistent episodes of excessive drowsiness in the daytime, or exaggerated, extended nighttime sleep
Hyp/ Hypo	lacking, situated below or underneath	**Hypo**spadias	a congenital defect in male infants, where the urethral opening is situated on the penis's underside
Idio	singular, isolated	**Idio**syncrasy	pertains to a rare and unpredictable individualized sensitivity to the effects of a pharmaceutical substance
Intra	inside, into	**Intra**venous catheter	a catheter inside a vein/ inserted into a vein
Mac-ro	large	**Macro**mastia	hypertrophy of the breasts

Micro	small	**Micro**aspiration	Accidental aspiration of tiny amounts of refluxed gastric content into the lungs
Post	succeeding, after, located behind	**Post**prandial	after a meal
Pre	prior, former, before, situated in front of	**Pre**prandial	before a meal Thus, preprandial glucose level pertains to your glucose level before you eat.
Semi	half	**Semi**conscious	the individual is only partially cognizant of his surroundings
Syn	linked	**Syn**drome	where a cluster of symptoms are linked by a single causative agent
Trans	from side to side, through	**Trans**orbital	passing through the eye socket
Ultra	extreme, beyond normal	**Ultra**sound	sound waves that travel at an extremely high frequency (vibrations that are higher than 20,000 per second)

Medical Antonyms

It is easy to decode the definition of a medical term if you know how to spot the prefix. Prefixes like Hyper and Dys are so common in everyday language, that once you get to identify them in medical terms, the convoluted term tends to seem less daunting.

Another useful trick to avoid confusion is to keep your eyes peeled for negative counterparts. Some medical terms may have the same root words and may initially look or sound the same. However, a change in a letter here or there can completely transform the meaning of the word.

Prefix	Meaning	Example of the Meaning	Meaning of the Example
Ab	to move away from	**Ab**duction	a movement away from the body's midline
Ad	to move toward	**Ad**duction	a movement toward the body's midline
Bio	life	**Bio**psy	when a tissue obtained from a living body is examined to determine the existence, the cause, or the severity of an illness
Necro	death	**Necro**psy	when a pathologist examines a dead body to determine the deceased's cause of death
Brady	Slow	**Brady**pnea	abnormally slow breathing, usually under 12 breaths per minute

Tachy	fast	**Tachy**pnea	abnormally rapid breathing, more than 25 breaths per minute
Endo	in	**Endo**genous depression	biologically based depression, not caused by external factors
Exo	out	**Exo**genous depression	depression caused by a causative factor outside the body (eg: the environment, other people, events)
Eu	regular, well	**Eu**thymia	a mood that is normal and rationally positive
Dys	hard, irregular, not well	**Dys**thymia	a mild, albeit persistent type of depression
Hyper	too much, more than	**Hyper**plasia	the enlargement of an organ or tissue caused by an increase in the reproduction rate of its cells.
Hypo	too little, less than	**Hypo**plasia	under-development or incomplete development of a tissue or organ It refers to an insufficient or below-normal number of cells.

Retro	backward	**Retro**grade amnesia	Type of memory loss where the person can no longer access events that happened in the past, specifically ones before the occurrence of an injury or disease
Ante-ro	Forward	**Antero**grade amnesia	the inability of the affected individual to form new memories following the event which caused the memory loss

Medical Synonyms

In the medical language, there is a tendency for several words to have the same meaning. Part of the reason is because a huge chunk of medical terms, including prefixes, were derived from Greek and Latin tongues. Hence, it's possible for a modern medical prefix to have both a Greek version and a Latin version which may be used by healthcare professionals interchangeably.

Take a look at the following identical prefixes in their Greek and Latin forms.

Body Part	Greek	Latin
Kidneys	**Nephro** **Nephro**lithiasis the formation of stones in the kidneys	**Ren/ Reno** **Ren**al failure other term for kidney failure
Navel	**Omphalo** **Omphalo**phobia an irrational fear of belly buttons	**Umbilico** **Umbilico-**plasty surgical procedure to repair or augment the belly button
Teeth	**Odont/ Odonto** **Odonto**blast refers to a cell in the tooth germ which manufactures dentin	**Dent/ Dento** **Dent**al abscess buildup of pus in the gums or the teeth
Breast	**Mast/ Masto** **Mast**ectomy surgical excision of the breast/s	**Mamm/ Mammo/ Mamma** **Mammo**plasty surgical procedure to augment the breast/s

Medical Terminology

Words meaning dual/ both
Ambi **Ambi**dexterity the ability of a person to carry out manual tasks with either hand with equal competence
Bi **Bi**fid uvula two clefts in the uvula
Di **Di**gastric muscle muscle under the jaw consisting of two bellies

More Synonymous Prefixes

Words meaning bad, faulty, difficult, or painful
Dys
Dyspepsia
ineffective digestion
Mal
Malabsorption
inability of the small intestinal lining to absorb essential nutrients

Words meaning against
Anti
Antidote
a substance which works by contradicting the action of a toxic substance
Contra
Contraceptive
a device or a drug which acts against the normal mechanisms which lead to conception

Medical Terminology

Words meaning above
Epi **Epi**gastric situated above the stomach
Super **Super**ciliary bony prominence above the sockets of the eyes/ pertaining to the eyebrow
Supra **Supra**sternal situated above the sternum

Words meaning under
Infra **Infra**patellar below the knee
Hypo **Hypo**glossal below the tongue
Sub **Sub**lingual below the tongue

Prefixes Pertaining to Position and Direction

Prefix	Meaning	Example of the Meaning	Meaning of the Example
Cir-cum	around	**Circum**cision	a surgical procedure wherein the foreskin con-cealing the tip of the penis is removed

A circumferential incision is made around the pe-nis's tip.

While often done for hygienic or religious reasons, it may also be performed as a treatment for balanitis, which is the inflammation of the head of the penis. |
| Dia | Through | **Dia**thermy | a procedure wherein heat is produced in the body through high frequency electric current.

It may be done as a treatment for ischemia to boost blood flow to the area. It may also be performed to alleviate pain that originates deep in the body. |
| In | inside, into | **In**tubation | a procedure wherein a tube is inserted into a body cavity or an anatom-ical part |
| Inter | Between | **Inter**stitial | situated between a body part or cells, such as in the case of **inter**stitial fluid |

Intra	within	**Intra**vascular fluid	pertains to fluid contained within blood vessels It consists primarily of serum, in which blood cells are suspended.
Juxta	alongside, near	**Juxta**-anasto-mic artery	refers to the artery situat-ed just before the area of anastomosis
Meso	in the middle	**Meso**derm	pertains to the middle layer of the skin
Para	alongside, beyond, two similar parts	**Para**uterine	near the uterus
Peri	around	**Peri**auricular	around the outer ear
Pre	prior to, be-fore, situated in front of	**Pre**operative	before surgery
Pro	situated in front of, prior to	**Pro**gnosis	knowledge gathered beforehand It pertains to a scientific estimate of the most probable outcome of a disease.
Re	back	**Re**gurgitation	commonly used to de-scribe the backward flow of undigested food matter back into the esophagus or the mouth It may also be used to describe the backflow of other fluids, including blood.
Opist-ho	situated behind, retro-grade	**Opistho**tic	the bony elements behind the inner ear's capsule

Prefixes for Numbers and Measurements

Prefix	Meaning	Example of the Meaning	Meaning of the Example
Deci	one tenth	**Deci**bel	means one tenth of a 'bel' It is a unit used to express the relative intensity of sound.
Kilo	means 1000	**Kilo**gram	a unit of mass, equivalent to a thousand grams
Milli	means one thousandth	**Milli**osmole	1/1000 of an osmole
Mono	means one	**Mono**cyte	a cell with one nucleus
Nulli	zero	**Nulli**para	pertains to a female who has had no children
Primi	first	**Primi**gravida	pertains to a female on her first pregnancy
Quadri	means four	**Quadri**plegia	when all four extremities are paralyzed
Semi	half	**Semi**circular	half circle or half encircling, as in the case of the **semi**circular canal These are bony spaces in the inner ear that are filled with fluid. They are crucial in maintaining balance and in providing the brain with facts about orientation.

Tetra	four	**Tetra**cyclic antidepres-sants	antidepressant drugs with four fused atom rings in their skeletal formulas Includes Mirtazapine and Mianserin
Tri	three	**Tri**cyclic anti-depressants	antidepressant drugs with three atom rings in their chemical structures Includes Amitriptyline and Doxepin
Uni	one	**Uni**cellular	pertains to a cell with one nucleus

Note: Some measurement prefixes do not pertain to a specific number. Rather, they are used as comparative accessories to distinguish the abnormal from the normal.

An example of such prefix is **Poly** like in **Poly**dipsia. This is an unusually great and insatiable thirst experienced as a symptom of a disease (eg: Diabetes)

The Most Important Suffixes

Below is a table of the most indispensable suffixes in the medical field accompanied by their meanings and examples of their applications.

Suffix	Meaning	Example of the Meaning	Meaning of the Example
Cyte	a cell	Erythro**cyte**	red blood cell
Cytosis	pertains to cells and their functions	Phago**cytosis**	refers to the process wherein a cell swallows up (phago) a particle like a microorganism, a foreign substance, or an old blood cell This is part of the normal immune function of the body.
Esis	pertains to a condition, sometimes refers to a disease process or a symptom It may not always give a word a negative meaning.	Enur**esis** / Encop**resis**	the clinical terms for bedwetting and for fecal incontinence
Ion	suggests an action	Circumduc-**tion**	pertains to the circularl (round and round) motion of an extremity
Spasm	an involuntary muscular contraction	Broncho-**spasm**	paroxysms of the smooth muscles which cause the bronchi to constrict

Stasis	ceasing/ re-maining at a constant level	Chole**stasis**	a condition wherein there is a blockage of bile flow from the liver to the small intestines
Steno-sis	constricting or narrow-ing of an anatomical passage	Aorto**steno-sis**	when the aorta narrows due to: congenital causes, because of wear and tear (in geriatric patients), or when the person has suffered from rheumatic fever in the past and the aortic valve is scarred
Tion	could pertain to either a process or a state	Diges**tion**	the process of breaking food down mechanical-ly and with the aid of enzymes, to convert them into substances that are beneficial to the body
Toxic	poisonous to	Hema**toxic**	pertains to something which is poisonous to the blood
Uria	refers to the state of the urine, often abnormal	Hemat**uria**	the presence of blood in the urine
Y	pertains to a state or a condition, sometimes positive and sometimes negative	Dactyl**y**/ Syndactyl**y**	While the former pertains to the arrangement of the fingers and toes, the latter is a term used to refer to adhesions between two or more of the digits

Suffixes for Surgical and Diagnostic Procedures

Suffix	Meaning	Example of the Meaning	Meaning of the Example
Cente-sis	a sterile procedure done to remove fluid from an anatomical cavity or space	Amnio**centesis**	a procedure where the amniotic sac is surgically punctured, so that the doctor can obtain a fluid sample
Clasis	to crush	Osteo**clasis**	In this corrective procedure, a bone is intentionally fractured by the surgeon in order to repair a deformity.
Desis	fusion done through an operative procedure	Artho**desis**	In this procedure, a joint is immobilized after its surface is fused with that of an adjacent bone.
Ectomy	pertains to the surgical excision or removal of a tissue, an organ, or an anatomical part	Thyroid**ecto-my**	the surgical removal of a diseased or toxic thyroid gland
Graphy	a diagnostic procedure where X-ray or CT images are produced and recorded	Angio**graphy**	examination by X-ray or CT of blood or lymph vessels, carried out after the introduction of a radiopaque substance

Gram	a procedure which could pertain to writing, recording, or using X-ray films for diagnostic purposes	Cardio**gram**	In this method, the muscle activity in the heart is recorded with the use of a cardiograph.
Graph	pertains to a tool used to record or to create X-ray images for diagnostic use	Cardio**graph**	a device used to evaluate the health status of the heart It is capable of detecting discrepancies in the electrical potential, which stimulates heartbeat.
Meter	a measuring instrument	Sphygmoma-no**meter**	This device is used to measuree blood pressure.
Metry	refers to the process of obtaining measurement	Pelvi**metry**	where the dimensions of a pregnant woman's pelvis are measured, in relation to the delivery of an infant
Opsy	means to check or to examine	Bi**opsy**	the removal of a sample tissue from the body of a patient so it can be examined under a microscope
Pexy	a reparatory surgical procedure	Sacrocol-po**pexy**	the surgical repair of slackened organs of the pelvis
Plasty	operative reconstructive procedure for therapeutic or cosmetic purposes	Rhino**plasty**	the clinical term for correction of nasal deformities

Rrha-phy	patching tissues up with sutures	Nephro**rrha-phy**	a surgical technique wherein a detached kidney is kept in place by stitching it into the posterior abdominal wall It is also a term used for repair of an injured kidney.
Scope	any instrument designed to allow visual examination of an anatomical cavity or an organ of the body	Oto**scope**	a tool used to examine the ear canal and the eardrum visually
Scopy	refers to the process of assessing an organ or a cavity of the body visually, with the aid of an instrument	Rhino**scopy**	a procedure done to look at the interior of a patient's nose by inserting a rhinoscope (a tube with light and a lens) directly into the patient's nasal cavity
Stomy	surgical method of establishig a new opening in the body	Sigmoid**osto-my**	the creation of a secondary anus through a stoma (opening) via the sigmoid colon
Tomy	to cut	Phlebo**tomy**	using a needle for gaining access into a vein This is for the purpose of drawing blood.

Suffixes for Pathological Conditions

Suffix	Meaning	Example of the Meaning	Meaning of the Example
Algia	pain	Arthr**algia**	clinical term for joint pain
Asthenia	lack of strength	My**asthenia** Gravis	is a severe autoimmune neuromuscular disorder which is manifested by an unpredictable degree of weakness of the body's voluntary muscles
Cele	pertains to an herniation or the protrusion of a body organ	Cysto**cele**	is the herniation of the bladder into the weakened vaginal wall
Dynia	pertains to pain	Gastro**dynia**	stomach pain
Ectasia/ Ectasis	dilatation which occurs in a hollow body organ	Lymphangi**ec-tasia**	when a lymph vessel is dilated due to an external cause (such as a blockage in the local lymphatic drainage)
Edema	a condition wherein excessive fluid accumulates in the tissues of the body, or in a body cavity	Cephalo**edema**	Refers to edema that occurs within the head, due to fluid buildup

Emesis	the clinical term for vomiting	Pye**mesis**	the vomiting of pus
Emia	pertains to a blood condition	An**emia**	a clinical condition characterized by red blood cell or hemoglobin deficiency The affected individual suffers from pallor and fatigue.
Ia	a condition	Insomn**ia**	a persistent condition wherein the affected individual is unable to sleep
Iasis	suggests an abnormal or unhealthy state	Elephant**iasis**	a parasitic infection which is manifested by severe swelling of the extremities The causative agent is the filarial worm which may be transferred between human beings via a female mosquito bite. The parasite develops into a grown worm, which dwells in the affected individual's lymphatic system.
Ism	indicates a condition of	Priap**ism**	persistent and painful penile erection, that occurs even without external and psychological stimulation
Itis	inflammation	Col**itis**	when the lining of the colon is inflamed

Lith	suggesting the presence of a calculus or a stone, may also mean resembling a stone	Feca**lith**	when a mass of feces is stuck into the intestinal tract and hardens, so that it resembles a stone
Lysis	breakdown, death of	Electro**lysis**	the breakdown of structures, such as a cancerous mass, through electric currents
Lytic	decomposition of, inhibition of, annihilation of	Anxio**lytic**	Pharmaceutical drug prescribed to deter anxiety
Megaly	the abnormal enlargement of	Cardio**megaly**	the disproportionate enlargement of the heart This could be due to the excessive thickening of the heart muscle, or it could be brought about by the expansion of one or more of the heart chambers.
Malacia	softening/ weakening of	Bronchoma-**lacia**	when the cartilaginous wall of the bronchial tubes become floppy or weak This commonly occurs in babies less than six months of age.

Oma / Ma	indicative of malignancy, an abnormal mass, a tumor	Retino**blasto-ma**	a malignant form of eye cancer wherein immature cells rapidly develop in the retina This is occurs in young children, and is caused by gene mutation in the chromosomes.
Osis	suggests a condition or a state, often an abnormal one	Halit**osis**	an unpleasant odor from breath, due to poor hygiene, or as a symptom of a clinical condition
Pathy	indicates a disease or dysfunction	Neuro**pathy**	when one or more of the peripheral nerves are dysfunctional, causing the affected individual to become weak or numb
Penia	lack of	Granulocyto-**penia**	a significant decrease in the number of gran-ulocytes The latter are white blood cells which are essential in the immune functions of the body. They contain granules, which are actually microscopic pouches, which carry enzymes that digest microbes.

Phobia	extreme sensitivity to, irrational fear of	Photo**phobia**	severe sensitivity to light, which may be brought about by an infection (such as Rabies), trauma to the eye, or as an effect of a procedure (cataract surgery)
Plegia	meaning paralysis	Cyclo**plegia**	a condition wherein the ciliary muscle of the eye is paralyzed
Ptosis	the downward displacement or drooping of an anatomical part	Uvulo**ptosis**	also known as a falling palate This is a condition wherein the uvula relaxes and elongates.
Rrhage/ Rrhagia	the abnormally excessive flow of, rupture of	Hemo**rrhage**	the profuse leakage of blood from a vessel
Rrhea	excessive flow of a bodily discharge	Dia**rrhea**	the passage of loose, watery stools, several times more than usual
Rrhexis	the rupture of a body organ or a vessel	Angio**rrhexis**	when a blood vessel becomes ruptured
Sclerosis	hardening of	Athero**sclerosis**	A condition in which there is fatty plaque deposits in the inner walls of the arteries, causing them to harden

Grammatical Suffixes

» There are some medical suffixes which, when attached to a root word, form an adjective. Some serve to refer to a body system, an anatomical organ, a process, or a condition.

Ac/ Ar/ Ary/ Eal/ Ic/ Al/ Ous/ Tic
Cardi**ac** – pertaining to the heart
Ventricul**ar** – of the ventricle/ connected to the ventricle
Pulmon**ary** – part of the lungs/ originating from the lungs
Esophag**eal** – from the esophagus/ part of the esophagus
Allerg**ic** – brought about by an allergy
Intestin**al** – belonging to or connected to the intestines
Eczemat**ous** – related to eczema
Therapeu**tic** – concerning therapy

» There are also suffixes which, when added to a word, changes its meaning from a noun to a verb

Ize/ Ate
Anesthet**ize** – to provide anesthetic, hence to cause loss of sensation or consciousness
Lact**ate** – the act of producing milk
Coagul**ate** – to congeal or to solidify fluid such as blood

*The latter may also be used to refer to a result of a process or an offshoot of something

Ate
Opiate – an opium derivative
Hemolysate – an offshoot of hemolysis

» Occasionally, you may come across flexible suffixes with various meanings.

When the suffix **Genic** is added to a root word, this may mean "caused by".

Ex: Cocci**genic** means produced by cocci

However, sometimes, -genic could also be used to mean "causing".

Example: Colla**genic** which means that it triggers the production of collagen

Another use of -genic is to indicate association with a gene. Ex: Tri**genic**

» Suffixes are often used to suggest the characteristics, the purpose, or the ability of something.

Ory	Ile
Sens**ory** - used for perception, feeling, or sensing (e.g. Sens**ory** neurons)	Erect**ile** - possessing the ability to become erect Contract**ile** - creates contractions

The above suffixes are, at times, also used to indicate a connection to a body system, an anatomical organ, or a disease process.

Aud**ile** – concerning the auditory nerves

Respiratory – connected with the organs for respiration (e.g. Respiratory muscles)

Moreover, **Ile**, in itself may be used to indicate a condition.

E.g: *A patient is febrile when he has a body temperature that is above normal.*

> » **Oid** is a suffix which is used to suggest the resemblance of something to another.

Mucoid for instance, means something which resembles mucus.

> » Some suffixes are used to signify specialties or specialists in the medical field.

Ician pertains to a professional in a specific field of study.

A Pediatrician is a specialist in the field of medicine dealing with child health and with treating children's illnesses.

Trics relates to medicine, doctors, or treatment.

Obstetrics is a branch of medicine which deals with childbirth and with caring for mothers who are about to give birth, are giving birth, or have given birth.

Iatry is from the Greek word 'iatrea' which translates to "the art of healing". This suffix pertains to a medical profession.

Podiatry is a branch of medicine concerned with the health and treatment of the illnesses and infections of the human foot.

Ian, on the other hand, is used to refer to an expert in a field of study.

An example of this is a Geriatrician, who deals with elderly people.

Ist is a suffix used to denote a certified practitioner, such as in the case of a Pharmacist who possesses a license to dispense pharmaceutical drugs.

Ologist is affixed to a word to pertain to someone who concentrates in a specific field of study. A Psychologist specializes in psychology. However, only a Psychiatrist is licensed to prescribe medications to patients.

Ology, of course, means study, as in Neurology

This is a field of medicine that is concerned with the parts, the working, and the disorders of the nervous system and the nerves.

» There are suffixes which are attached to nouns to emphasize their singular form.

Um	Us
The Cerebell**um** is the part of the brain located in the rear of the skull. It governs vital functions, such as coordination and muscular movement.	A Streptococc**us** is a single bacterium.

» Lastly, there are suffixes which, when added, to a root word, has a diminutive effect.

Icle	Vesicle	a small sac filled with fluid
Ole	Arteri**ole**	the tiniest branch in the arterial circulation
Ula	Mac**ula**	tiny pigmented patches on the skin without elevation
Ule	Pap**ule**	Clinical term for a small pimple or a raised swelling on the skin It may be inflamed, but it is not pus-filled.

Ready for an exercise now?

Medical Terms Exercise

Instruction: Choose the right answer.

1. Suffix "uria" is? **Answer:** _____
   - condition of urine
   - urethra
   - kidney
   - ureter

2. Amyl/o is? **Answer:** _____
   - gland
   - fat
   - male
   - starch

3. Prefix "ab" is? **Answer:** _____
   - down
   - away from
   - up
   - towards

4. Prefix "polio" is what color? **Answer:** _____
   - black
   - yellow
   - gray
   - red

5. Suffix "oid" is? **Answer:** _____
   - away
   - resembling
   - different
   - middle

6. Onc/o is? **Answer:** _____
   - growth
   - tumor
   - cell
   - nail

7. Prefix "neo" is? **Answer:** _____
   - child
   - old
   - baby
   - new

8. Narc/o is? **Answer:** _____
   - death
   - stupor
   - night
   - drug

9. Suffix "lithiasis" is? **Answer:** _____
   - presence of stones
   - crushing
   - narrowing
   - presence of fluid

10. Prefix "hemi" is? **Answer:** _____
    - quarter
    - tenth
    - half
    - cut

11. Ot/o is? **Answer:** _____
    - ear
    - bone
    - auricle
    - ossicle

12. Splen/o is? **Answer:** _____
    - spleen
    - spasm
    - pulse
    - sternum

13. Suffix "natal" is? **Answer:** _____

    - pregnancy
    - woman
    - birth
    - new

14. Prefix "chlor" is? **Answer:** _____

    - blue
    - black
    - green
    - white

15. Prefix "retro" is? **Answer:** _____

    - past
    - present
    - forward
    - backward

Great job! Answers are in the second to the last chapter.

Chapter 7:

Eponyms, Homonyms, and More

Homonyms

Derived from the Greek term *Homonymos* which translates to "same name", homonyms refer to words which are pronounced in the same (or in almost the same) way. However, they have completely different definitions. Their spellings may also differ.

The English language is stuffed with homonyms, and so is the medical language. Thus, when healthcare workers communicate with each other, or with their patients, it becomes necessary to check, recheck, and keep rechecking prescriptions, requests, orders, verbal reports, etc. just to make sure that one was able to understand the other correctly. Even if you're not in the medical field, it would be advantageous to know whether your doctor is talking about the long bone in your forelimb (humerus) or if he just thinks you're funny (humorous).

In the table below, you'll find a compilation of the most common, most slippery medical homonyms.

Agonist	Antagonist
a pharmaceutical agent that triggers the action of cell molecules in a manner that they would be stimulated by the naturally occurring byproducts	an element which neutralizes, obstructs, or combats the action of another

Anuresis the inability of the affected individual to pass urine	**Enuresis** uncontrolled urination especially while sleeping at night
Apophysis A part of a bone that juts out	**Epiphysis** the rounded edge of a long bone
Aural pertaining to the ear, its parts, and its functions	**Oral** pertaining to the mouth, its parts, and its functions
Cor pertaining to the heart	**Core** the midpoint
Diaphysis a long bone's shaft situated between the epiphyses **Diathesis** an individual's predisposition to a certain health condition	**Diastasis** a condition wherein anatomical parts that are usually joined together end up separating; may occur in bones as well as muscles
Dyskaryosis anomalous change in the squamous epithelial cell manifested as an irregular nuclear structure; may precede the formation of a malignant neoplasm	**Dyskeratosis** unusual keratinization (hardening of the protein in the skin, hair, and nails) which occurs in cells under the granulous layer of the epidermis
Dysphagia trouble with swallowing	**Dysphasia** diminished ability to comprehend speech, due to brain injury or a disease

Galactorrhea uncharacteristic flow of milk from the breasts	**Galacturia** milky coloring of the urine
Humeral concerned with the humerus	**Humoral** concerned with body fluids
Hypophysis pertains to the pituitary gland	**Hypothesis** a scientific supposition, which seeks to provide an explanation for a phenomenon
Ileum the third region of the colon, situated between the cecum and the jejunum	**Ilium** the broadest region of the pelvic bone
Lice ectoparasites which can infest various hair-bearing parts of the body, from the head to the toe	**Lyse** to destroy
Malleolus the bony projection in the ankle that resembles a mallet	**Malleus** a mallet-shaped bone in the middle ear
Metaphysis pertains to the broad part at the tip of a long bone	**Metastasis** when a secondary malignant growth develops away from the initial site of the cancer
Mucous mucus-secreting, such as in mucous membranes	**Mucus** sticky secretions secreted by mucous membranes, that act as a protectant and a lubricant

Medical Terminology

Osteal that which resembles, affects, involves, or is related with the skeleton	**Ostial** pertains to an os/ostium (which in medical terms, means opening)
Profuse copious such as in profuse bleeding	**Perfuse** to bring about the flow or the dissemination of something within a tissue
Radicle the smallest subdivision in a nerve	**Radical** created to get rid of every possible prolongation or spread of a morbid process, such as in radical treatment
Resection when part of an anatomical structure or organ is surgically removed	**Recession** a surgical procedure of the eye, done to correct strabismus (improper alignment of the eyes)
Tract may pertain to a normal anatomical system of organs such as the respiratory tract It may also be used to refer to an aberrant passage through the tissue, such as in the case of a fistula which just creates a deviant system of its own	**Track** pertains to a route, such as in Z track injection
Vesicle a tiny fluid-carrying sac, like the seminal vesicles of men	**Vesical** pertains to the bladder
Viscus the single form of viscera, meaning internal organ	**Viscous** viscid, gelatinous, used to describe bodily secretions

Eponyms

From the Greek word *eponymos* which translates to "to name", Eponyms in medical terms refer to the person, object, or place after which a disease, an instrument, a clinical sign, or a procedure was named. It's a great way to honor the doctors, the scientists, or the researchers who have discovered, designed, inspired, improved, or invented these tools, methods, and knowledge that we are using today.

Medical Term	Named After...	Meaning
Achilles Tendon	a hero in Greek mythology who was physically invulnerable, except for a part of his heel	also referred to as the calcaneal tendon, located at the back part of the leg. It is the thickest tendon in the human anatomy.
Addison's disease	Dr. Thomas Addison who was the first one to identify the condition in the 1950's	a potentially life-threatening disease, brought about by incompetent adrenal glands, that are incapable of producing sufficient levels of cortisol
Allis clamp	Oscar Huntington Allis who introduced it in the 1880's	a surgical clamp used for holding soft tissues, that is still extensively used today
Alzheimer's Disease	German Neurologist Alois Alzheimer	a worsening deterioration of the mental faculties, caused by brain degeneration. The affected individual experiences memory loss, as well as a decline in his cognitive abilities.

Apgar Score	its inventor, Virginia Apgar, who was a specialist in the field of Obstetrics	an efficient and quick way to conduct initial assessment of a neonate's health after it is born
Bartholin's Gland	Caspar Bartholin the Second, who discovered it in the 17th century	two small glands situated on either side, and slightly behind the vaginal opening These glands are responsible for secreting mucus to provide lubrication to the vaginal region.
Bell's palsy	surgeon and neurologist Charles Bell	paralysis of the facial nerve, which renders the affected individual incapable of controlling the muscles on the affected side of the face.
Broca's Aphasia	Paul Broca, a French anatomist and surgeon	inability of the affected person to create complete sentences, or to join words together This is due to the damage sustained by the left front part of the brain after a stroke.
Cushing Syndrome	Harvey William Cushing	a series of symptoms brought about by excessively elevated levels of cortisol Along with other symptoms, the affected individual experiences weight gain and thin skin that is easily bruised.

Down's syndrome	John Haydon Down, an English doctor in the 1800's	Also referred to as trisomy 21, it is a chromosomal disorder in which affected children manifest characteristic physical features. It is accompanied by delayed physical and mental development, with some degree of learning disability.
Eustachian Tube	Italian anatomist, Bartolomeo Eustachi, who discovered it	also referred to as the auditory tube, it serves as a connection between the middle ear and the nasopharynx
Heimlich Maneuver	American surgeon, Henry Heimlich	In emergency medicine, this abdominal thrust is performed during choking to rid the airways of obstruction by a foreign body.
Hodgkin's lymphoma	British physician Thomas Hodgkin who made the first account of this disease in the 1830's	a malignant lymphoma characterized by night sweats, a febrile condition, loss of weight, and enlarged albeit painless lymph nodes These may be palpated in the neck, in the axilla, or in the groin.
Homans' Sign	an American surgeon called John Homans	When pain is experienced in the calf region upon dorsiflexion of the foot, this is referred to as Homans' sign. It is indicative of deep vein thrombosis.

| Whipple's Procedure | Allen Whipple | an upper gastrointestinal surgical procedure where the head of the pancreas adjacent to the duodenum is removed

This is performed as a treatment for cancer of the pancreas.

The duodenum is removed as well, along with certain areas of the gallbladder and the common bile duct.

Sometimes, in this radical procedure, a portion of the stomach is also taken out. |

Acronyms

Medical acronyms are abridged versions of medical terms. They are usually made up of the initial letters or syllables of the full term. Sometimes, these acronyms are written in uppercase but that may not always be the case.

Every day, people use words that they don't even realize were actually acronyms. These include *radar* which actually stands for Radio Detection and Ranging. That's because such words have become so deeply integrated into everyday life that eventually, the letters just gave birth to a new word. The same truth applies to the medical field. The following are the most frequently encountered acronyms in the medical language.

Acronym	Meaning
AF	Atrial Fibrillation
AIDS	Acquired Immune Deficiency Syndrome
ARDS	Acute Respiratory Distress Syndrome
BPH	Benign Prostatic Hyperthropy
CAT scan	Computerized Axial Tomography
CNS	Central Nervous System
COPD	Chronic Obstructive Pulmonary Disease
CSF	Cerebrospinal Fluid
CVA	Cerebrovascular Accident
CXR	Chest X-ray

Medical Terminology

ECG	Electrocardiogram
ECT	Electroconvulsive Therapy
EEG	Electroencephalogram
ET	Endotracheal Tube
FB	Foreign Body
FHR	Fetal Heart Rate
GERD	Gastroesophageal Reflux Disease
GI	Gastrointestinal
HR	Heart Rate
HRT	Hormone Replacement Therapy
IBD	Inflammatory Bowel Disease
IBS	Irritable Bowel Syndrome
ICU	Intensive Care Unit
IUD	Intrauterine Device
KVO	Keep Vein Open
MRI	Magnetic Resonance Imaging
MS	Multiple Sclerosis
MVA	Motor Vehicle Accident
NG	Nasogastric
NSAID	Non-Steroidal Anti Inflammatory Drug
PEA	Pulseless Electrical Activity

PID	Pelvic Inflammatory Disease
PPIs	Proton Pump Inhibitors
PT	Prothrombin Time
SZ	Seizure
TAH	Total Abdominal Hysterectomy
THR	Total Hip Replacement
TKR	Total Knee Replacement
UA	Urinalysis
V/Q SCAN	Ventilation Perfusion Scan
VTACH/ VT	Ventricular Tachycardia

Abbreviations

In the medical field, time is definitely gold. The survival, safety, and wellbeing of a patient does not just depend on how properly care is provided, but also on how *promptly* it is delivered. Thus, it is essential that professionals in the medical field create an efficient style of communication that is as quick as it is thorough. Being clear and concise is the key. For this reason, healthcare industry professionals make use of abbreviations. Below are the most commonly encountered abridgements in the medical area and what they mean.

frequently used in relation to pharmaceuticals

a.c. means prior to meals so the drug ordered a.c. will have to be administered before feeding. Conversely, **p.c.** is to be taken after meals.

b.i.d. means two times daily however, if a drug is to be taken strictly every 12 hours, then q12 is written.

cap is a shorter term for capsule.

gtt means drops, commonly used when ordering IV fluids.

IM is short for intramuscular and it usually pertains to the route of injection.

K means potassium. Potassium with chloride is **KCL**.

Meanwhile, sodium is **Na**. Both electrolytes are essential to the body's functions and thus, healthcare workers tend to keep an eye on their levels when a patient is under intensive care.

O.D is the condensed form of right eye while **O.S.** means left eye. To pertain to both eyes, **O.U.** is used. These are important especially when administering prescribed eye treatments like opthalmic drops.

PR is per rectum. This means a PR drug, such as a suppository, is to be administered rectally.

When a physician writes down **q.d.**, it means that a drug must be taken every day. **qod**, on the other hand, means every other day. **q.i.d** is four times daily.

*These do not just pertain to drugs but also to other interventions. (ex. chest therapy q.i.d. means to provide physiotherapy to the patient four times a day)

q2h and **q3h** mean every 2 hours and every 3 hours respectively.

qAM, **qPM**, and **qhs** stands for every morning, every evening, and every each bedtime correspondingly.

STAT means that the order must be carried out immediately.

frequently used in relation to surgery and treatment

BKA means below the knee amputation

A **DNR** order means Do Not Resuscitate. Hence, when a patient goes into cardiac arrest, the medical team will not take any measures to resuscitate him. This is applicable to near death patients wherein the priority is to ensure a peaceful and dignified passing.

Rather than saying "in the body", a quicker way to do it would be to say **in vivo**.

In vitro, on the other hand, means in the laboratory, as in the case of In Vitro Fertilization.

LLQ stands for left lower quadrant. The definition of this will be discussed more thoroughly in the succeeding chapters.

Meanwhile, **LUQ** is left upper quadrant.

npo is the abbreviation for nil per oral or nothing by mouth. This means that a patient is not allowed to consume food or drinks prior to or after a surgical procedure or a diagnostic test.

RLQ means right lower quadrant. So if a patient is complaining from pain in the right side of the abdomen, specifically in the lower region, then the medical professional can write down RLQ pain or pain in RLQ.

RUQ means right upper quadrant.

tab refers to medication in tablet form.

frequently used in relation to assessment, documentation, and diagnostics

a/g refers to the ratio of albumin to globulin

BP pertains to blood pressure

C&S means culture sensitivity test; a test performed to identify a pathogen, and to determine the best choice of medicine that can be used to inhibit its growth

CC is an abbreviation for chief complaint. This indicates the reason why the patient sought medical attention in the first place. (ex: CC of fever for 7 days)

This is not to be confused with cc in small letters. **cc** stand for cubic centimeters, customarily used when measuring the amount of fluid taken from a patient's body.

CBC stands for complete blood count. This blood test is conducted to assess a person's general health. It is effective in detecting a broad range of hematological and non-hematological disorders.

When a physician writes down **D/C**, this means something (a treatment, a drug, etc.) will have to be discontinued.

On the other hand, **DC** means discharge and is used to indicate that the patient is ready to go back home from the hospital.

DTR means Deep Tendon Reflexes. This is what the doctor checks for when s/he hits a tendon with a hammer.

DOE is short for Dyspnea On Exertion. This means a patient may not be having difficulty of breathing while he's at rest but he is dyspneic when he's ambulatory or performing activities.

DX stands for diagnosis.

LBP is lower back pain

N/V is the abridged form of nausea and vomiting.

T is temperature as measured by a thermometer.

frequently used in relation to diseases
DM is short for diabetes mellitus
DVT means Deep Vein Thrombosis (when a blood clot occurs in a deep vein/s of the body. The leg is the most affected body part.)
FX indicates a fracture
HTN stands for hypertension
Upper respiratory tract infections and urinary tract infections are common enough to warrant their own abbreviations: **URI** and **UTI**

Symbols

Why do medical professionals bother with symbols? It's not that they are deliberately trying to be cryptic. Actually, the reason why symbols are used for communication in the medical setting is because they tend to speed things up. A nurse can easily understand a doctor's order just by glancing at an icon, thus saving precious time.

Moreover, symbols also help in preventing confusion between healthcare professionals. This is especially true in cases where words can be interpreted differently by various individuals. Simply put, symbols are more likely to provide uniformity and are less prone to personalized, biased interpretation.

Medical Terminology

In the medical language, another way to write **Approximate** is ≈.
α is **Alpha** so instead of jotting down alpha adrenergic blockers, you can put down α-blockers.
A shorter way to say **At** is @.
Meanwhile, this symbol means **Before**: ā
Δ means **To Change**.
When describing **Degrees**, a healthcare professional may just put down **1o**, **2o 3o**, which means first, second, and third degrees respectively.
↑ means **Increase** or **Increased**. Hence, to advise a patient to increase consumption of liquids, the physician may write ↑ fluid intake.
Correspondingly, ↓ means **Decrease** or **Decreased** such as in ↓ urine output. (decreased urine output)
A **Female** subject may be represented by ♀. Just as a **Male** subject may be signified by ♂.
Just like in basic math, < in Medicine means **Less than** and > means **Greater than**.
Likewise, = means **Equal to**.
Instead of writing down **None**, you can put down Ø.
50 **Micrograms** of a drug is 50 **μg**.
+ pertains to **Positive** whereas – means **Negative**.

Chapter 8:

Pluralizing Medical Terms

Rules for the Formation of Plurals

When it comes to the formation of plural forms in the medical language, the following general rules apply:

> » If the singular form of the word ends in an **–a** suffix, then it is written in the plural form by adding an **e** at the end.

E.g: bursa = bursa**e**

> » If the singular form of the word ends in an **–ex** suffix or in an **–ix** suffix, then it is changed into the plural form by turning the ending into **–ices**.

E.g: apex = ap**ices**

> » That said, if the singular word ends in **-nx**, such as in the case of phalanx, then the x is removed and changed to **ges**.

E.g: phalanx = phalan**ges**

> » Still, if the singular form of the words ends only with an **-x**, then the plural form is created by replacing x with **ces**.

E.g: thorax = thora**ces**

» When it comes to pluralizing singular words ending in –**is**, the end i is changed into an **e**.

E.g: testis = test**es**

There are,, however, certain exceptions:

Epididymis is changed into epididym**ides**.

Femoris is pluralized into femor**a**.

Iris in its plural form is ir**ides**.

» If the singular form of the medical term ends with an **-on**, replace the last two letters with **a**.

E.g: ganglion = gangli**a**

» The same rule applies to singular medical words ending in -**um**.

E.g: labium=labi**a**

» To pluralize singular words ending in -**us**, just remove the us and then add **i**.

E.g: malleolus = malleol**i**

There are, however, a few exceptions to this rule:

Corpus is changed into corp**ora**.

Plexus in its plural form is plexus**es**.

Viscus is pluralized into visc**era**.

» In the medical vocabulary, there are lots of terms ending in –**itis**. To change these into plural form, remove the itis and then affix **itides**.

E.g: meningitis = mening**itides**

» Meanwhile, singular words than end in –**is** are changed into the plural form dropping the is and placing **ides** in its stead.

E.g: arthritis = arhrit**ides**

» For singular medical terms that end in **-y**, the plural form is made by using **ies** to replace the y.

E.g: biopsy = biops**ies**

» For singular words ending in **-yx**, remove the x and replace with **c**. Afterwards, add **es**.

E.g: calyx= caly**ces**

» There are singular words that end in **ma/ oma**. In such cases, **ta** is added.

E.g: sarcoma = sarcoma**ta**

» There are also medical terms in which the singular and the pluralized forms are the same.

E.g: meatus = meatus

» How are medical terms that consist of two words dealt with? Easy. If the words were derived from Latin, and if they are a combination of a noun and an adjective, change both words into the plural form.

E.g: placenta previa = placenta**e** previa**e**

» Inevitably, there are a handful of terms which seem to be immune to all these rules.

Cornu is pluralized into cornu**a**.

Vas in its plural form is vas**a**.

Pons is changed into pon**tes**.

More Rules in the Medical Language

>> When the medical word is of English origin, apply the rules that your grammar teacher taught you. To pluralize words, the end is simply changed to **s**.

E.g: infection = infection**s**

>> However, if the word ends in **-s**, add **es**.

E.g: stress = stress**es**

>> The same rule applies to English medical terms ending in **-ch**.

E.g: crutch = crutch**es**

>> The previous rule also goes for English medical words ending in **-x** or in **-sh**.

E.g:

wash = wash**es**

flex= flex**es**

>> If the singular English medical term ends in **-y**, see if the y is preceded by a consonant. If yes, then change the y to **i**. Then, add **es**.

E.g: palsy = pals**ies**

>> If the singular English medical term ends in **o**, see if the o is preceded by a consonant. If yes, add **nes**.

E.g: comedo = comedo**nes**

Exceptions to the rule include embryo, which is pluralized to embryo**s** and placebo in which the plural form is placebo**s**.

>> As mentioned previously, abbreviations are used daily in the medical setting. As a general rule, measurement abbreviations are immune to the rules stated above.

E.g:

While one might say that *the cervix is a few centimeters dilated*, one cannot say that *the cervix is 3 cms dilated*. That's because the latter already comes with a number value.

Thus, the proper sentence would be: **The cervix is 3 cm dilated.**

> » Numbers with single digits are pluralized by adding **'s** (s with an apostrophe).

E.g: The patient was asked to count backwards by 2**'s**.

That said, the apostrophe is dropped when pluralizing numbers with two digits and above.

Wrong: The patient is in his late 40's.

Correct: **The patient is in his late 40s.**

> » When it comes to pluralizing acronyms, simply add an **s** to terms written in uppercase.

E.g: The abridgment for white blood cell is WBC.

To write white blood cells, put down WBC**s.**

> » That said, if an abbreviation is written in the lowercase, then an apostrophe is needed.

E.g: wbc = wbc**'s**

Chapter 9:

The Structure and Organization of the Body

Anatomical Planes

Anatomical planes refer to imaginary perpendicular and parallel lines drawn across the body, to divide it into sections. For medical professionals, this makes description of specific areas of the body easier.

» **Coronal Plane**

This is otherwise known as the Frontal Plane. It is the vertical place which separates the human body into anterior and posterior portions.

» **Midsagittal Plane**

This is also referred to as the body's midline. It is a horizontal plane which separates the left side of the body from the right, and vice versa.

» **Sagittal Plane**

This refers to a vertical plane which goes from the anterior to the posterior part of the body while separating the body into left and right portions.

» **Transverse Plane**

This pertains to a cross-wise plane which is parallel to the ground, and passes through the waistline. It separates the upper half of the human body from the lower half.

Body Positions

The following are the most commonly encountered terms which describe the position of the body as a whole.

» **Anatomic Position**

This is when the human body is standing upright. The arms are lying at each side and the palms are faced forward. Feet are positioned side by side and the toes are pointing forward.

» **Erect**

When the subject is standing upright.

» **Genupectoral**

Also referred to as the knee-chest position, it is when a patient goes on his knees on an examination table/bed. Then, his head and the upper part of his body are lowered onto the table/bed.

In this position, the majority of the body's weight is carried by the chest and the knees. This is preferable for rectal examinations.

» **Lateral Recumbent**

A side-lying position (either left or right) where the knee of one leg is slightly bent.

» **Sims Position**

A side-lying position wherein the patient is lying on his left side, but his right thigh and his right knee is pulled up toward his chest.

» **Prone**

When the patient is lying face down, and flat on his abdomen.

» **Dorsal Recumbent**

When the subject is lying flat on his back, facing up. (also known as supine)

» **Lithotomy**

The patient starts off in the supine position. Then, with the thighs apart, the legs are drawn towards the abdomen.

» **Fowler**

The patient lies supine, but the head part of the bed is raised 18 inches and the patient's knees are elevated.

» **Trendelenburg**

A position in which the subject is lying on his back, with the legs at a higher level than the head..

Body Regions

To most patients, a tummy ache is a tummy ache. However, if a patient can provide the healthcare professional with information as to which specific part of the abdomen is in pain, s/he can have an idea as to which internal body organs may be involved.

To make diagnoses easier and more accurate, the abdominal area is divided into four separate regions.

The Four Regions of the Abdomen

» **RUQ**

This is the right upper quadrant. In it, you'll find the right lobe of your liver along with your gallbladder, a portion of the small intestine, and a portion of the large intestine.

» **LUQ**

The left upper quadrant of the abdomen houses the stomach. It also contains the left lobe of your liver. In it, you'll find vital organs such as the pancreas and the spleen. It also contains portions of the small intestine and part of the large intestine.

» **RLQ**

In the right lower quadrant, you'll find the appendix. It also contains areas of the small and the large intestines. At the same time, it holds the right side of the ureter. In females, it houses the right ovary and the right fallopian tube.

» **LLQ**

Accordingly, the left lower quadrant contains the left ovary and the left fallopian tube in females. It also holds the left ureter. Moreover, it contains portions of the small intestine and parts of the large intestine.

The Nine Regions

The abdominal-pelvic areas are further divided into nine subdivisions.

Region	Location	Body organs
Region I **Right Hypochondriac Region**	found in the upper right part of the abdomen, specifically underneath the lower rib cartilage	the gallbladder the liver's right lobe
Region II **Epigastric Region**	situated in the middle of the two hypochondriac regions, specifically in the superior part of the abdomen and below the lower rib cartilage	some of the right lobe of the liver, some of the left lobe of the liver, a huge portion of the stomach
Region III **Left Hypochondriac Region**	in the upper left part of the abdomen, specifically under the lower rib cartilage	a tiny part of the stomach, some parts of the large intestine
Region IV **Right Lumbar Region**	found in the abdomen's mid-section, under Region I	parts of the large intestine, parts of the small intestine
Region V **Umbilical Region**	in the abdomen's mid-section, specifically in the middle of the two lumbar regions, under Region II	some of the transverse colon, some of the small intestine
Region VI **Left Lumbar Region**	situated in the mid-left abdominal area, under Region III	some of the small intestine, a portion of the colon
Region VII **Right Inguinal Region / Right Iliac Region**	lower right part of the abdomen, under Region IV	some of the small intestine, the cecum

Region VIII **Hypogastric Region**	mid-lower part of the abdomen, under Region V	the urinary bladder, the appendix, part of the small intestine
Region IX **Left Inguinal Region/ Left Iliac Region**	found in the lower left abdominal area, below region VI	some of the colon, some of the small intestine

The Five Regions of the Spinal Column

The spinal column is also segmented into five different regions. This table describes these regions, from the top to bottom.

Region	Abbreviation	Vocabulary	Location	Details
Cervical Region	C	Cervic/o = Neck	neck area	this forms the bones of the neck and is composed of seven vertebrae, labeled as C1 to C7
Thoracic Region	T or D	Thorac/o = Chest	in the chest area	This consists of the vertebrae in the chest region, and is composed of 12 vertebrae, labeled as T1 to T12 (or D1 to D12) Each of these bones is connected to a rib.

Lumbar Region	L	Lumb/o= Loins	found in the flank part, situated between your hip bone and your ribs	comprises of four vertebrae, labeled as L1 to L5 They make up the movable part of the spine. The vertebrae in this region are considered to be the strongest and largest of all.
Sacral Region	S	Sacr/o = Sacrum	below the lumbar vertebrae	consists of five vertebrae labeled from S1 to S5 As a child matures, these bones fuse together to create one big bone, which is the sacrum.
Coccygeal region	Co	Coccyx = tailbone	situated at the lowermost end of the vertebral column	initially made up of four mini bones, Co1 – Co4, which fuse together before adulthood to create one small bone

The Smaller Regions Found in the Body

Region	Location
Auricular	situated around the ears
Axillary	the armpits
Buccal	the inner part of the cheeks (facial)
Clavicular	on either side of the breastbone
Infraorbital	located below the eye/s
Infrascapular	The region at the back of the body, just below the scapula (shoulder), on either side of the vertebrae.
Interscapular	in the posterior part of the body, between the shoulder blades
Lumbar	The lower part of the back, inferior to the infrascapular area
Mammary	spans the area all over the breast/s
Mental	around the chin
Orbital	around the eye/s
Pubic	inferior to the pubis
Sacral	over the sacrum
Sternal	over the sternum
Submental	under the chin
Supraclavicular	above the clavicles

Body Cavities

The human body consists of two major cavities, which are then divided into smaller cavities. These are hollow spaces which serve to shelter the internal body organs.

Ventral Cavity

The ventral cavity houses the internal organs located in the anterior part of the body. The following table shows its subdivisions.

Sub-cavity	Vocabulary	Organs
Thoracic Cavity	Thorac/o = Chest	This sub-cavity carries vital organs such as the lungs, the heart, and the aorta. In this cavity, you'll also find the esophagus and the trachea.
Abdominal Cavity	Abdomin/o = Abdomen	Vital internal organs contained in this sub-cavity are the stomach, the intestines, the liver, and the kidneys. The abdominal cavity also contains the spleen, the gallbladder, and the pancreas.
Pelvic Cavity	Pelv/i = Pelvis	Contained in this sub-cavity are the reproductive organs. It also houses the urinary bladder.

Dorsal Cavity

This major cavity carries the internal organs found in the posterior side of the body.

Sub-cavity	Vocabulary	Organs
Cranial Cavity	Crani/o = Skull	This sub-cavity cradles the brain.
Spinal Cavity	Spin/o = Spine	In this sub-cavity, you'll be able to locate the spinal cord, and nerves arising from it.

Body Parts

View these tables to find out which medical terms correspond to specific body parts.

Anterior	
Antebrachial	Forearm
Antecubital	Inner elbow
Axillary	Armpit
Brachial	Arm
Carpal	Wrist
Celi/o	Abdomen
Cephalic	Head
Cranial	Cranium
Crural	Leg
Facial	Face

Medical Terminology

Frontal	Forehead
Femoral	Thigh
Inguinal	Groin
Mammary	Breast
Ocular	Eye
Oral	Mouth
Palmar	Palm
Patellar	Kneecap
Pedal	Foot
Phalangeal	Fingers/ Toes
Pubic	Pubis
Tarsal	Toes
Thoracic	Chest
Umbilical	Navel

Posterior	
Cervical	Neck
Gluteal	Buttock
Iliac	Hip
Lumbar	the lower part of the back
Occipital	the base of the skull
Parietal	the crown of the head
Popliteal	the back of the knee
Sacral	Sacrum
Scapular	Shoulder
Tarsal	Ankle
Plantar	the sole of the foot

Chapter 10:

Terminology of Body Systems

As you've read earlier, one of the most effective techniques in memorizing and decoding medical terms is to group them according to body systems. In this chapter, you'll find the most important root words associated with each major system of the body along with examples of their usage.

The Cardiovascular System			
Root Word	Meaning	Example of the Meaning	Meaning of the Example
Angi/ Angio	pertaining to a blood vessel	**Angio**ma	a non-malignant tumor of the blood vessel wall
Aort/ Aorto	pertaining to the aorta which is the largest artery in the human body	**Aort**itis	a condition where the aorta is inflamed

Arter/ Ateri/ Arterio/ Artero	pertaining to an artery Arteries are the vessels which carry oxygenated blood from the heart.	**Arter**iole	a smaller blood vessel which braches out from an artery
Ather/ Athero	pertaining to fatty substance	**Ather**oma	occurs when damaging fatty matter accumulates in the inner layer of the arterial walls
Atri/ Atrio	pertaining to the atrium, which can be either one of the two superior heart chambers	Cavo**atrial** junction	The point where the vena cava and the upper wall of the right atrium of the heart meet
Cardi/ Cardio	pertaining to the heart	**Cardio**logist	a specialist who focuses on the health and the diseases of the heart and the blood vessels
Hemangi/ Hemangio	pertaining to blood vessels	**Hemangi**oma	an anomalous mass of blood vessels
Pericardi/ Pericardio	pertaining to the pericardium, which is the protective sheath enveloping the heart	**Pericardio**centesis	the aspiration of fluid from the pericardial sac

Phlebo	relating to the veins	**Phlebo**lith	a tiny calcification inside a vein
Thromb/ Thrombo	pertaining to blood clot	**Thrombo**cytes	blood components which serve to prevent bleeding through clotting
Vas/ Vaso	related to blood vessel	**Vaso**depressors	pharmaceutical agents which decrease blood pressure by creating a relaxing effect on the blood vessels

Medical Terminology

The Respiratory System			
Root Word	**Meaning**	**Example of the Meaning**	**Meaning of the Example**
Alveol/ Alveolo	pertains to the alveoli, which are air sacs found at the end of the bronchioles	**Alveol**itis	when the alveoli are inflamed
Bronch/ Bronchi/ Broncho/ Bronchio	pertaining to the bronchi, which are the two air passages from the trachea to the lungs	**Broncho**pneumonia	bacterial, viral, or fungal infection of the lungs, originating from the bronchi
Capn/ Capno	relating to carbon dioxide	**Capno**meter	a device which is used to monitor and measure the carbon dioxide concentration of a patient's exhaled air.
Epiglott/ Epiglotto	pertaining to the epiglottis, which is a cartilagenous flap that provides a covering to the larynx during swallowing. This way, the food will not enter the airway.	**Epiglott**itis	when the epiglottis is inflamed

Laryng/ Laryngo	Pertaining to the laryx or the voice box	**Laryngo**malacia	the weakening of the larynx This rare condition occurs in neonates.
Mediastin/ Mediastino	pertains to the mediastinum which is the median part of the thoracic cavity	**Mediastin**al Shift	occurs when the organs which make up the mediastinum move toward the other side of the thoracic cavity
Nas/ Naso	pertains to the nose	**Naso**labial folds	the clinical term for laugh lines which run from the nose down to the corner of the mouth
Ox/ Oxi/ Oxo/ Oxy	pertains to oxygen	Pulse **Oxim**eter	a device used to monitor and measure the oxygen saturation of the blood via an indirect method
Pleur/ Pleuro	pertains to the pleurae which are dual layers of membrane that are located on the outside of the lungs	**Pleur**itis	when the pleura is inflamed

The Gastrointestinal System			
Root Word	**Meaning**	**Example of the Meaning**	**Meaning of the Example**
Append/ Appendo/ Appendic	pertaining to the appendix	**Appendic**olith	hardened deposits in the appendices
Bil/ Bili/ Bilo	pertaining to bile, which is the yel-low-brownish to green-like fluid that the liver secretes, and keeps in the gallbladder Its purpose is to aid in the digestion of fat.	**Bili**ary ob-struction	a blockage in the bile ducts
Cec/ Ceco	pertains to the cecum, which is a sac located over the large intestine, and joined to the ileum's bottom part. The ileum is the bottom-most part of the small intestine.	**Cec**ostomy	a surgical pro-cedure in which a catheter is inserted into the cecum

Dueden/ Duodeno	pertaining to the duodenum, which is the topmost part of the small intestine, where semi-digested food matter mixes with bile and other intestinal juices	**Duoden**itis	when the duodenum is inflamed
Esophag/ Esophago	relating to the esophagus	**Esophag**eal varices	dilated veins in the esophagus
Gastr/ Gastro	pertaining to the stomach	**Gastro**plasty	Surgical procedure wherein the size of the stomach is reduced, to make it smaller This procedure is used as a last resort for management of morbid obesity.
Sial/ Sialo	pertaining to the saliva	**Sial**adenitis	A condition in which the salivary glands are inflamed.

The Endocrine System			
Root Word	**Meaning**	**Example of the Meaning**	**Meaning of the Example**
Aden/ Adeno	gland	**Aden**opathy	a disease in the glands
Adren/ Adreno/ Adrenalo	pertains to the hormone-producing adrenal gland	**Adreno**megaly	abnormal overgrowth of the adrenal gland
Gluc/ Gluco	related to glucose	**Gluc**agon	a hormone secreted by the pancreas, which increases blood glucose levels
Glyc/ Glyco	pertains to glycogen, which is a compound used to store glucose. It is kept in the liver, until required for future energy purposes	**Glyco**genesis	the process wherein glucose is converted into glycogen
Gonad/ Gonado	pertains to the sex glands	**Gonado**tropin	a hormone responsible for aiding in the growth of gonads (reproductive endocrine glands, which create sex cells)
Pancreat/ Pancreato	pertains to the pancreas	**Pancreat**ectomy	the surgical removal of the pancreas

Parathyroid/ Parathyroido	pertains to the parathyroid gland, which is responsible for maintaining normal levels of calcium in the blood	Hypo**parathyroid**ism	severely reduced levels of parathyroid hormone in the blood This leads to calcium deficiency, which can in turn cause abnormal spasms of the muscles.
Thyr/ Thyro	pertaining to the thyroid gland, which is responsible for regulating the metabolic functions of the body	**Thyro**toxicosis	excessive amounts of thyroid hormone

	The Integumentary System		
Root Word	**Meaning**	**Example of the Meaning**	**Meaning of the Example**
Adipo	pertaining to fat	**Adipo**sis	disproportion-ate accumu-lation of fat in the body, or in an organ.
Derm/ Dermo/ Dermato	relating to the skin	**Dermo**phytosis	when the skin, hair, or nails are infected by a type of fungus that thrives in dead keratin.
Hidr/ Hidro	pertaining to sweat	**Hidro**cystomas	cystic growths in the apocrine sweat glands
Kerat/ Kerato	scaly tissue	**Kerat**osis	skin lesion, in which there is a coating of scaly tissue on the skin surface.
Lip/ Lipo	fatty	**Lipo**suction	the surgical removal of un-wanted excess fat, by inserting tubes beneath the skin
Melan/ Melano	black	**Melano**ma	A pigmented tumor contain-ing melano-cytes.

Myc/ Myco	concerning fungi	**Myco**sis	any infection with a fungus as a causative agent eg. candidiasis
Onych	nail	**Onycho**my-cosis	when the nails are infected by fungi
Seb/ Sebo	pertaining to the sebum or to the seba-ceous glands	**Sebo**rrhea	a condition where there is an abnormally profuse sebum production due to overactive sebaceous glands
Steat	pertaining to fat	**Steat**itis	when the fatty tissues are inflamed
Trich/ Tricho	related to hair	**Tricho**mycosis	infected condi-tion of the hair shaft, caused by fungi.

The Musculoskeletal System			
Root Word	**Meaning**	**Example of the Meaning**	**Meaning of the Example**
Humer/ Humero	pertaining to the humerus	**Humer**oulnar joint	It is a joint in the arm consisting of the humerus and the ulna bones.
Ili/ Ilio	relating to the ilium	**Ilio**femoral	concerning the ilium and the femur
Ischi/ Ischio	pertaining to the ischium	**Ischio**rectal abscess	an abscess created by the accumulation of pus between the rectum and the ischium
Kyph/ Kypho	bent	**Kypho**sis	when the spine is curved outward, such as in hunchbacks
Lamin/ Lamino	pertaining to the lamina (thin, flat area on either side of the vertebra's arch)	**Lamino**plasty	an operative procedure done toy relieve the pressure off the spinal cord, in order to treat spinal stenosis
Leiomy/ Leiomyo	smooth muscle	**Leiomyo**ma	a smooth muscle tumor, that is non-malignant
Lumbo	referring to the five vertebrae located on the lower back	**Lumbo**tomy	when the kidney is excised from the back

Maxill/ Max-illo	pertaining to the upper jaw	**Maxillo**lacri-mal	concerning the maxilla and the lacrimal bone
My/ Myo	muscle	**Myo**sitis	when the muscle tissue is severely inflamed, and prone to degeneration
Oste/ Osteo	relating to the bone	**Oseteo**arhtir-itis	arthritis which results due to the wearing of cartilage, causing bones to rub against each other. This is typically accompanied by pain in the bone and the joint.
Scolio	curved	**Scolio**sis	a condition wherein the spine is abnormally curved sideways
Spondyl/ Spondylo	pertaining to the vertebra	**Spondyl**itis	when the vertebra is inflamed
Synov/ Synovo	relating to the synovial membrane, which is a connective tissue that lines the joint cavities This produces synovial fluid, which provides lubrication to joints.	**Synov**itis	when the synovial membrane of the joint is inflamed

The Nervous System			
Root Word	**Meaning**	**Example of the Meaning**	**Meaning of the Example**
Cerebell/ Cerebello	pertains to the cerebellum, the major brain division that governs musculoskeletal movement	**Cerebell**itis	the inflamed state of the cerebellum
Cerebr/ Cerebro/ Cerebri	pertains to the cerebrum, the major part of the brain that governs feelings, behavior, memory, and thoughts	**Cerebr**algia	pain in the head, mainly associated with the meninges
Crani/ Caranio	pertaining to the cranium	**Cranio**tomy	a hole that is made surgically in the skull
Mening/ Meningo/ Meningio	concerning the meninges	**Meningi**oma	a tumor, usually non-malignant, that occurs in the brain's meningeal tissues
Neur/ Neuri/ Neuro	relating to a nerve	**Neuro**transmitters	chemicals that trigger the transition of signals from one nerve cell to another

The Sensory System			
Root Word	**Meaning**	**Example of the Meaning**	**Meaning of the Example**
Audi/ Audio	pertains to hearing	**Audio**metry	the measurement of an individual's sense of hearing, both in terms of sensitivity and range
Cochle / Cochleo	pertaining to the cochlea of the ear	**Cochle**ostomy	a surgical procedure wherein an opening is made in the cochlea
Conjunctiv/ Conjunctivo	referring to the conjunctiva of the eye	**Conjunctiv**itis	when the mucous membrane that lines the eyelid (conjunctiva) is inflamed
Cor/ Core/ Coreo/ Coro	pertaining to the pupil of the eye	**Coreo**plasty	corrective surgical procedure to fix the shape or the size of the pupil
Corne	relating to the cornea, the transparent front part of the eyeball which bends light	**Corne**al abrasion	a scratch in the outer layer of the cornea
Cycl/ Cyclo	pertaining to the ciliary body of the eye	**Cyclo**tropia	a kind of strabismus (clinical term for cross-eye)

Dacry/ Dacryo	tears	**Dacryo**cystitis	infected lacrimal sac/s
Larcrim/ Lacrimo	tears	**Lacrim**otomy	a surgical incision made into the lacrimal duct. The lacrimal glands work to keep the eyes moist. They are also responsible for the production of tears.
Scler/ Sclero	pertaining to the white of the eye	**Scler**astasia	protrusion of the sclera

Chapter 10: Terminology of Body Systems

The Urinary System			
Root Word	**Meaning**	**Example of the Meaning**	**Meaning of the Example**
Cyst/ Cysto	concerns the bladder, the organ where urine is collected prior to its excretion from the body	**Cysto**pexy	a surgical procedure wherein the urinary bladder is attached to the abdominal wall, or to other adjacent structures
Glomerul/ Glomerulo	pertaining to the glomerulus These are a group of capillaries found in the functional part of the kidney (the nephron).	**Glomerulo**ne-phritis	condition where the glomeruli are inflamed
Meat/ Meato	pertaining to a meatus (an external opening, eg. the urethra)	**Meat**otomy	pertains to a surgical procedure wherein the meatus is enlarged
Nephr/ Nephro	refers to the kidneys	**Nephro**calci-nosis	a condition wherein calcium salts are deposited in the renal parenchyma. This is one of the many undesirable consequences of hyperparathyroidism.

Pyel/ Pyelo	pertains to the renal pelvis (area in the center of the kidney where urine is collected)	**Pyelo**gram	an X-ray inspection of the kidneys, the bladder, and the ureters with the aid of a contrast medium introduced into veins
Ren/ Reno	concerning the kidneys	**Reno**megaly	abnormal overgrowth of the kidney
Ureter/ Uretero	pertains to the ureter, which is either one of the two ducts that transport urine from the kidney towards the urinary bladder	**Ureter**ostomy	a surgical procedure wherein an opening is created within the ureter, so that the flow of the urine can be diverted away from the bladder This is done in the case of a dysfunctional or surgically excised bladder.
Urethr/ Urethro	relating to the urethra, the conduit through which urine is transported from the bladder to be eliminated from the body	**Urethr**ostomy	the surgical creation of a permanent opening in the urethra, for the purpose of removing stones or other structures that are blocking the flow of urine

Chapter 10: Terminology of Body Systems

The Female Reproductive System			
Root Word	**Meaning**	**Example of the Meaning**	**Meaning of the Example**
Cervic/o	referring to the cervix	**Cervic**itis	when the cervix is inflamed
Colp/ Colpo	pertaining to the vagina	**Colpo**rrhagia	excessive vaginal bleeding
Galact/ Galacto	milk	**Galacto**cele	a cyst in the mammary gland, that contains milk
Gynec/ Gyneco	concerns the female reproductive parts	**Gynec**oid pelvis	the normal shape of the female pelvis
Hyster/ Hystero	pertaining to the uterus	**Hystero**salpingogram	an X-ray exam performed to determine the patency (freedom from obstruction) of the fallopian tubes
Lact/ Lacto	involving milk	**Lacto**genic	a substance, such as a drug or a hormone, which triggers milk production
Oo	egg	**Oo**genesis	refers to the process by which the ovum forms, develops, and reaches maturity

Oophor	pertaining to the ovaries	**Oophor**itis	when the ovaries are inflamed
Ovari/ Ovario	involving the ovaries	**Ovario**hyster-ectomy	the surgical excision of the ovaries, along with the uterus
Perine/ Per-ineo	relates to the perineum, which is the space that sep-arates the labia majora from the anus	**Perineo**meter	a device used to measure the strength of the muscular con-tractions of the pelvic floor
Vulv/ Vulvo	pertains to the vulva	**Vulv**itis	when the vulva is inflamed

The Male Reproductive System			
Root Word	**Meaning**	**Example of the Meaning**	**Meaning of the Example**
Andro	relates to males	**Andro**gen	a hormone which triggers and maintains male character-istics
Balan/ Balano	pertains to the head of the penis (glans penis)	**Balano**pos-thitis	the inflam-mation of the head of the penis and the foreskin

Epididym/ Epididymo	relates to the epididymis, which are clusters of sperm-storing ducts, located over the testes	**Epididymo**va-sostomy	a surgical procedure wherein a disconnected vas deferens is connected to the epididymis The vas deferens refer to a slender tube where sperm is transported from the epididymis to the urethra.
Orch/ Orchi/ Orchid/ Orchio	pertains to the testes	**Orchid**ectomy	a surgical procedure in which the testes are removed
Prostat/ Prostato	involves the prostate gland	**Prostat**itis	inflamed condition of the prostate
Sperm/ Spermo/ Spermato	concerning sperm	A**sperm**ia	a condition wherein the male is unable to produce semen

Chapter 11:

Answers

This section contains answers to exercises from the previous chapters.

A. Answers to Chapter 3

1. laryng
2. neur
3. oste
4. cardia
5. encephal
6. peri - itis
7. pathy
8. electro - gram
9. hyper - emia
10. rhin
11. bone
12. hypotension
13. true
14. false
15. Colonoscopy

B. Answers to Chapter 4

1. j
2. guy
3. j
4. f
5. k
6. sk
7. k
8. f
9. e
10. new
11. e
12. see
13. si
14. f
15. thee

C. Answers to Chapter 6

1. condition of urine
2. starch
3. away from
4. gray
5. resembling
6. tumor
7. new
8. stupor
9. presence of stones
10. half
11. ear
12. spleen
13. pregnancy
14. green
15. backward

Chapter 12:

Tips and Additional Resources

Every week, millions of viewers tune in to television shows about doctors, and delight at the medical language onscreen "doctors" use. Fans pick up bits and pieces of medical terms and assume they're now wise and knowledgeable about medical language. It's fun, but in truth, knowing and memorizing medical terms is not easy. There are millions of words to know and remember. Knowing where words came from and how they were formed is key. While everybody is not in the medical profession, and may not view medical-related shows, it is important to have at least a basic knowledge of medical terminology.

A. Tips

Here are some tips to help learners understand, pronounce, and memorize medical terms:

1. Build good study habits by taking down notes during class/training (when needed – it is still important to listen to instructors/teachers/ professors), organizing notes on lessons, and reading lessons regularly.

2. Rest when needed. Make sure to get enough rest because the human brain needs rest, too.

3. Create a schedule for studying. Choosing a specific time to study each day prevents cramming.

4. Ask for help when necessary, especially about lessons or medical terms that are really hard to understand. Classmates, professors, teachers, or instructors can always be approached for help.

5. Take practice tests or quizzes online. Many of them are interactive which takes boredom out of studying.

6. Play word games using flashcards, or other tools such as phone apps, or online interactive tools.

7. Aside from visual cues, learners can use other words that can be associated with medical terms. This is easier by using one's own words to describe a particular medical term. For example, inflammation of the nose is rhinitis. It can be associated with the word rhino.

B. Additional Resources

There are also other additional resources that can be used when studying medical terms, as follows:

1. Guides and Workbooks

Guides and workbooks are good alternatives to heavy medical dictionaries and books. The same information is provided when exploring them, but these are easier to understand, and are available in shorter versions. For instance, books that were written and developed to help learners understand medical terms and make them memorize words effectively.

Here are some of the best guides and workbooks for memorizing medical terms:

Medical Terminology: A Living Language

This book features a lot of medical information that are delivered for easy reading. It doesn't contain boring topics, usually seen in medical books. It also features up-to-date medical terms that were meticulously selected and cataloged. This book was written by Suzanne Frucht and Bonnie Fremgen.

Quick Medical Terminology: A Self-Teaching Guide

According to the authors, this book provides necessary tools for building and maintaining a large working knowledge of medical terms. They include a number of practice exercises, quizzes, and real examples to help learners develop and train their memory. This book was written by Shirley Steiner and Natalie Capps.

Medical Terminology for Dummies

This book is perfect even for non-medical professionals. It uses entertaining and engaging language to keep learners interested in learning medical terms. The book has managed to turn medicine from a serious field to something interesting and fun to read and learn. This book was written by Beverley Henderson and Jennifer Dorsey

2. Online Practice Quizzes

There are also a number of practice quizzes that are available online. Even some of the phone apps mentioned in Chapter 4 have their own online versions of their practice quizzes. These are fun to use because many of them are interactive. Some of the recommended online practice quizzes include:

Sporacle

This features a section dedicated to teaching medical terms, including hundreds of basic and complicated words. It offers addictive quizzes and timed exercises to keep learners interested.

ProProfs Quiz

This site also includes a section of quizzes that are related to medical terms and topics. It offers long quizzes with hundreds of questions.

3. Online Flashcards and Other Tools

Aside from quizzes and phone apps, there are also flashcards available online, that include games, exercises, and guides on how to create homemade flashcards. Some of the best online flashcards available are:

- » StudyBlue
- » Quizlet
- » StudyStack
- » Flashcard Machine

4. Free Online Classes

Lastly, there are online courses for learning medical terminology that are available for free. Anybody studying in medical training institutes or schools can still benefit from additional courses. They can add what they've learned from online classes to their knowledge base. Here are a few online programs that can be taken for free:

Medical Terminology Course

Provided by Des Moines University

This online course is divided into sections, and in each one are lessons containing practical and useful examples. Each lesson also includes additional information about topics being discussed, and there are quizzes and exercises at the end. Explanations are provided in an easy and light language and tone, which makes this online course easy to understand.

Medical Terminology

Provided by SweetHaven Publishing Services

This online class presents its lessons using flashcards. The class is divided into different modules that can be studied in a random order. Learners can pick any topic and work from there, which makes this online class perfect for busy medicals students, healthcare workers, and hospital personnel.

Understanding Medical Words

Supported by the National Library of Medicine

This online course can work even without Internet connection. It can be downloaded, so learners can review lessons offline. It offers a comprehensive list of medical terms with explanations and definitions. It also includes abbreviations most commonly used in the medical field. What's more, medical terms are broken down to their Latin and Greek roots. The course also provides examples with accompanying visuals.

These are just a few of many resources that can be added to a learner's arsenal of study tools. Now it's time to go and study.

Join Our Community

Medical Creations is an educational company focused on providing study tools for Healthcare students.

We want to be as close as possible to our customers, that's why we are active on all the main Social Media platforms.

You can find us here:

www.facebook.com/medicalcreations

www.instagram.com/medicalcreations

www.twitter.com/medicalcreation (no 's')

www.pinterest.com/medicalcreations

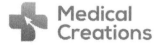

Conclusion

Thank you again for buying this book!

I hope this book was able to help you to better understand, memorize, and pronounce medical terms. The next step is to use the methods and tips provided here.

Finally, if you enjoyed this book, then I'd like to ask you for a favor, would you be kind enough to leave a review for this book on Amazon? It would be greatly appreciated!

Thank you and good luck!

Index

Index

Index

Hemiplagia, 68

Hemolysate, 92

Hemorrhage, 90

Hepatomegaly, 37

Heterochromia, 37

Hidrocystomas, 142

Histology, 38

Hodgkin's lymphoma, 105

Homan's sign, 105

Homeoplasia, 38

HR, 108

HRT, 108

HTN, 113

Humeral, 101

Humeroulnar joint, 144

Humoral , 101

Hydrocele, 38

Hyperhidrosis, 38

Hyperplasia, 71

Hypersomnolence, 68

Hypersplenism, 45

Hypochondriac, 124

Hypogastric , 125

Hypoglossal, 76

Hypoparathyroidism, 141

Hypophysis, 101

Hypoplasia, 71

Hypospadias, 68

Hypothesis, 101

Hypothyroidism, 46

Hysterectomy, 38

Hysterosalpingogram, 151

I

Iatrogenic, 39

IBD, 108

IBS, 108

ICU, 108

Idiosyncrasy, 68

Ileum, 101

Iliac, 124, 125

Iliac, 131

Iliofemoral, 144

Ilium, 101

IM, 110

In vitro, 111

In vivo, 111

Infraorbital, 127

Infrapatellar, 76

Infrascapular, 127

Inguinal, 124, 125, 130

Inguinodynia, 25

Index

P

Palatoplasty, 42

Palmar, 130

Pancreatectomy, 140

Papilloma, 28

Papule, 94

Parauterine, 78

Parietal, 131

Paronychia, 27

Patellar, 130

Pathogen, 42

pc, 110

PEA, 108

Pedal, 130

Pediatrician, 93

Pelvic cavity, 128

Pelviectasis, 28

Pelvimetry, 84

Percardiocentesis, 134

Perfuse, 102

Periauricular, 78

Perineometer, 152

Peritonitis, 42

Phagocytosis, 81

Phalangeal, 130

Phalloplasty, 28

Pharmacist, 93

Pharmacodynamics, 42

Pharyngitis, 43

Phlebitis, 43

Phlebolith, 135

Phlebotomy, 85

Photophobia, 90

Phrenic nerve, 43

Physiotherapy, 56

PID, 109

Pilocystic, 28

Plantar, 131

Pleurisy, 43

Pleuritis , 137

Pneumococcal, 56

Pneumothorax, 43

Podiatry, 29, 93

Poliomyelitis, 44

Polydipsia, 80

Popliteal, 131

Postprandial, 69

PPI, 109

Preoperative, 78

Preprandial, 69

Priapism, 87

Primigravida, 79

Index

Index

Viscus, 102

VT, 109

VTach, *see* VT

Vulvitis, 152

W

Whipple's procedure, 106

X

Xanthochromia, 48

Xerophthalmia, 48, 56

Z

Zika virus, 56

Kindle MatchBook

Kindle MatchBook is a feature that allows customers who have previously purchased a physical book from Amazon.com to receive the Kindle version for a discounted price or even for free.

You can receive a copy of our Medical Terminology Kindle Edition for FREE.

Just go to the Kindle Version page of the book on Amazon and download the ebook.

Read your ebook on any device (phone, tablet, laptop).

CHECK OUT OUR OTHER BOOKS

EKG/ECG Interpretation:
Everything you Need to Know
about the 12-Lead ECG/EKG
Interpretation and How to
Diagnose and Treat Arrhythmias

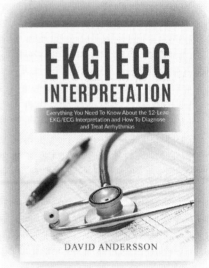

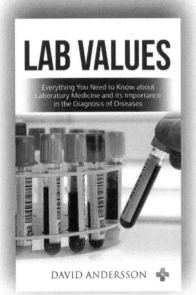

Lab Values: Everything You Need to
Know about Laboratory Medicine
and its Importance in the Diagnosis
of Diseases